**Omega–6/Omega–3 Essential Fatty Acid Ratio:
The Scientific Evidence**

World Review of Nutrition and Dietetics

Vol. 92

Series Editor

Artemis P. Simopoulos
The Center for Genetics, Nutrition and Health, Washington, D.C., USA

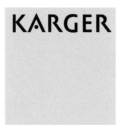

Omega–6/Omega–3 Essential Fatty Acid Ratio: The Scientific Evidence

Volume Editors

Artemis P. Simopoulos
The Center for Genetics, Nutrition and Health, Washington, D.C., USA

Leslie G. Cleland
Royal Adelaide Hospital, Adelaide, S.A., Australia

24 figures and 37 tables, 2003

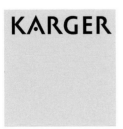

Basel · Freiburg · Paris · London · New York ·
Bangalore · Bangkok · Singapore · Tokyo · Sydney

············

Artemis P. Simopoulos
The Center for Genetics,
Nutrition and Health
Washington, D.C. (USA)

Leslie G. Cleland
Rheumatology Unit
Royal Adelaide Hospital
Adelaide, S.A. (Australia)

Library of Congress Cataloging-in-Publication Data

Omega–6/omega–3 essential fatty acid ratio : the scientific evidence / volume editors,
   Artemis P. Simopoulos, Leslie G. Cleland.
       p. ; cm. – (World review of nutrition and dietetics, ISSN 0084–2230 ; v. 92)
   Includes bibliographical references and index.
   ISBN 3–8055–7640–4 (alk. paper)
       1. Omega–6/omega–3 fatty acid ratio.   2. Essential fatty acids in human nutrition   I.
   Simopoulos, Artemis P., 1933–   II. Cleland, Leslie G.   III. Series.
       [DNLM: 1. Fatty Acids, Essential–metabolism.   2. Fatty Acids. Omega–3–metabolism.
   3. Linoleic Acids–metabolism. QU 90 O552 2003]
   QP752.E84O46 2003
   613.2′84–dc22

                                                                                    2003058871

Drug Dosage. The authors and the publisher have exerted every effort to ensure that drug selection and dosage set forth in this text are in accord with current recommendations and practice at the time of publication. However, in view of ongoing research, changes in government regulations, and the constant flow of information relating to drug therapy and drug reactions, the reader is urged to check the package insert for each drug for any change in indications and dosage and for added warnings and precautions. This is particularly important when the recommended agent is a new and/or infrequently employed drug.

© Copyright 2003 by S. Karger AG, P.O. Box, CH–4009 Basel (Switzerland)
www.karger.com
Printed in Switzerland on acid-free paper by Reinhardt Druck, Basel
ISSN 0084–2230
ISBN 3–8055–7640–4

....

Contents

V

Preface

Several sources of information suggest that human beings evolved on a diet with a ratio of omega–6 to omega–3 essential fatty acids of ~1 whereas in Western diets the ratio is 15/1–16.7/1, and in India ratios in urban areas range between 38/1 and 50/1 whereas in rural areas the ratios range from 5/1 to 6.1/1. Western diets are considered 'relatively deficient' in omega–3 fatty acids, because they contain excessive amounts of omega–6 fatty acids compared with the diet on which human beings evolved and their genetic patterns were established. Excessive amounts of omega–6 polyunsaturated fatty acids (PUFA) and a very high omega–6/omega–3 ratio, as is found in today's Western and Indian diets, promote the pathogenesis of many diseases, including cardiovascular disease, cancer, and inflammatory and autoimmune diseases, whereas increased levels of omega–3 PUFA (a lower omega–6/omega–3 ratio), exert suppressive effects. In the secondary prevention of cardiovascular disease, a ratio of omega–6/omega–3 of 4/1 was associated with a 70% decrease in total mortality. The same ratio of omega–6/omega–3 of 4/1 appears to be the optimal ratio for brain-mediated functions. A ratio of omega–6/omega–3 of 2.5/1 reduced rectal cell proliferation in patients with colorectal cancer, whereas a ratio of 4/1 with the same amount of omega–3 PUFA had no effect. The lower omega–6/omega–3 ratio in women with breast cancer was associated with decreased risk. A ratio of omega–6/omega–3 of 2–3/1 suppressed inflammation in patients with rheumatoid arthritis, and a ratio of 5/1 had a beneficial effect on patients with asthma, whereas a ratio of 10/1 had adverse consequences.

These studies indicate that the optimal ratio may vary with the disease or condition under consideration. This is consistent with the fact that chronic diseases are multigenic and multifactorial. Furthermore, genetic polymorphisms interact with the nutritional environment to define the phenotype. Therefore, it is quite possible that the therapeutic dose of omega–3 fatty acids will depend on the degree of severity of disease resulting from the genetic predisposition. A lower ratio of omega–6/omega–3 fatty acids is more desirable in reducing the risk of many of the chronic diseases of high prevalence in Western societies, as well as in the developing countries.

This volume on *Omega–6/Omega–3 Essential Fatty Acid Ratio: The Scientific Evidence* in the series *World Review of Nutrition and Dietetics* considers the scientific evidence of the importance of the omega–6/omega–3 essential fatty acid ratio in the prevention and management of a number of chronic diseases. Because the first person to consider the ratio was Ralph Holman, who also suggested the omega (ω) nomenclature, the 'omega (ω)' nomenclature was selected for this volume instead of the 'n-' nomenclature.

The volume begins with the paper on the 'Importance of the Ratio of Omega–6/Omega–3 Essential Fatty Acids: Evolutionary Aspects' by Artemis P. Simopoulos. The author considers the evidence and the factors that led to the excessive increases in the omega–6/omega–3 ratio. During evolution, the ratio of 18:2ω6 (linoleic acid, LA) to 18:3ω3 (α-linolenic acid, ALA) was 0.70/1 and the longer chain omega–6/omega–3 ratio was 1.79/1, just under 2. Therefore, from the evolutionary standpoint, the total omega–6/omega–3 ratio has a range of 1–2/1. Two countries' diets come close to the ratio of evolution: the traditional diet of Crete (Greece) and the traditional diet of Japan. In both countries, the rate of death due to cardiovascular disease is the lowest. It is now recognized that there is a need to return the omega–3 fatty acids into the food supply, both for normal growth and development and for the prevention and management of chronic diseases. In doing so, caution must be exercised to return the omega–3 fatty acids in type and amounts consistent with data obtained from: (1) studies on the evolutionary aspects of diet; (2) studies at the molecular level, and (3) data obtained from clinical intervention trials.

The second paper 'The Importance of Omega–6/Omega–3 Fatty Acid Ratio in Cell Function: The Gene Transfer of Omega–3 Fatty Acid Desaturase' by Jing X. Kang, is a confirmatory study at the molecular level of the omega–6/omega–3 ratio that supports the knowledge obtained from studies on the evolutionary aspects. In this paper Dr. Kang shows how the insertion of the missing delta-3 desaturase in cardiac myocytes and cancer cells in culture, leads to the production of 18:3ω3 from 18:2ω6, and eicosapentaenoic acid (EPA) formation from arachidonic acid (AA) proceeds until the ratio between omega–6 and omega–3 equals 1/1.

The next paper 'Omega–6/Omega–3 Ratio and Brain-Related Functions' by Shlomo Yehuda is a very extensive review of the evidence from experimental studies carried out in humans and rodents. Dr. Yehuda begins by discussing the evidence for the importance of the ratio and the relationship of essential fatty acids to the blood-brain barrier and the brain. He then describes the role of PUFA in brain neurotransmitters, membrane fluidity and myelin, prostaglandins, cholesterol and fatty acids and their influence on the fluidity index. Subsequently, he discusses the experimental studies on omega–3 fatty acid deficiency, PUFA and early development, the role of essential fatty acids in aging, Alzheimer's disease, fatty acid metabolism, and seizure control and multiple sclerosis. The effects of essential fatty acids on sleep showed that a ratio of 18:2ω6 to 18:3ω3 of 4/1 had beneficial effects in a group of students. The same ratio of 4/1 reduced the elevated levels of cortisol in rodents. Dr. Yehuda's review relates mainly to LA and ALA. The author concludes that a ratio of 18:2ω6 to 18:3ω3 of 4/1 is the optimal ratio of brain mediated functions.

Similarly, the paper 'Dietary Prevention of Coronary Heart Disease: Focus on Omega–6/Omega–3 Essential Fatty Acid Balance' by Michel de Lorgeril and Patricia Salen indicates that a ratio of 18:2ω6 to 18:3ω3 of 4/1 is associated with a decrease of 70% in total mortality from cardiovascular disease in a dietary pattern consistent with the diet of Crete in patients with one episode of myocardial infarction. The authors describe in detail the components of the diet, which is a modified diet of Crete, and their physiologic functions. Epidemiological studies as well as randomized dietary trials including moderate amounts of omega–3 fatty acids in the experimental diet suggest that these fatty acids, despite their low concentrations in blood and tissues, may be important in relation to the pathogenesis (and prevention) of coronary heart disease. Whereas a striking protective effect of an ALA-rich modified diet of Crete was reported with a 50–70% reduction of the risk of recurrence after 4 years of follow-up, it is still not known whether ALA is cardioprotective by itself only or also through its conversion into very long-chain omega–3 fatty acids (EPA and DHA) and then into the corresponding eicosanoids and prostaglandins. The authors state that, 'According to our current knowledge, dietary ALA should represent about 0.6–1% of total daily energy or about 2 g per day in patients following a Mediterranean type of diet, whereas the average intake of LA should not exceed 7 g per day. Supplementation with very long chain omega–3 fatty acids (about 1 g per day) in patients following a Mediterranean type of diet was shown to decrease the risk of cardiac death by 30% and of sudden cardiac death by 45%. Thus, in the context of a diet rich in oleic acid and poor in saturated and omega–6 fatty acids, even a small dose of very long chain omega–3 fatty acids (1 g in the form of capsules) might be very protective. These data underline the importance of the omega–6/omega–3 ratio in the prevention of coronary heart disease.'

In the next paper 'Effects of an Indo-Mediterranean Diet on the Omega–6/Omega–3 Ratio in Patients at High Risk of Coronary Artery Disease: The Indian Paradox,' Daniel Pella, Gal Dubnov, Ram B. Singh, Rakesh Sharma, Elliot Berry and Orly Manor clearly state that although the Indian diet is low in total fat, it has a high omega–6/omega–3 ratio of about 38/1, which is associated with high rates of cardiovascular disease and diabetes. Changing the cooking oils and increasing the fruit and vegetable intake in the diet brought the ratio down to 9.1/1 and a 40% decrease in cardiovascular disease mortality in both the primary and the secondary prevention of cardiovascular disease.

The paper 'Omega–6/Omega–3 Fatty Acid Ratio: The Israeli Paradox' by Gal Dubnov and Elliot Berry similarly points to the fact that nutrition habits in Israel include a low intake of energy, total and animal fat, combined with high levels of the hypolipidemic polyunsaturated fatty acids resulting in a seemingly healthy diet. Nonetheless, the prevalence of coronary artery disease, diabetes mellitus, and cancer in Israel is comparable to other Western countries, despite these dietary differences. The cause for this might be 'too much of a good thing', that is, too high levels of omega–6 polyunsaturated fatty acids, which may lead to insulin resistance, increased atherogenesis and thrombosis, coronary events and cancer. 'This is the Israeli paradox, reflecting the possible dangers of high omega–6 diet.'

Zampelas and co-workers in their paper on 'Linoleic Acid to Alpha-Linolenic Acid Ratio: From Clinical Trials to Inflammatory Markers of Coronary Artery Disease' review the protective role of ALA in cardiovascular disease, ALA's anti-inflammatory function, and their study on the effect of a ratio of LA/ALA of 1/1 in suppressing C-reactive protein (CRP). Their recent research suggests that a LA/ALA ratio of 1/1 could have an anti-inflammatory effect, by reducing interleukin-1β (IL-1β), IL-6, tumor necrosis factor-α (TNF-α), and CRP levels. Because the genes for IL-1β, IL-6, and TNF-α are polymorphic, the effects of ALA on their levels is dependent on the genetic variation of these cytokines.

Tomohito Hamazaki and Harumi Okuyama, in their paper 'The Japan Society for Lipid Nutrition Recommends to Reduce the Intake of Linoleic Acid: A Review and Critique of the Scientific Evidence' carried out a most thorough review and critique of the role of omega–6 and omega–3 polyunsaturated fatty acids in the prevention of coronary heart disease and other chronic diseases. The authors explain why 18:2ω6 should be reduced in the Japanese diet, which already has an omega–6/omega–3 ratio of 4/1. Their review clearly shows that LA intake should be reduced to 3–4% of energy. The Japanese have an omega–3 fatty acid intake of 0.6% of energy LNA and 0.5% of energy EPA and DHA. Their recommendation is consistent with an omega–6:omega–3 range of 2.7–3.6/1.

There is epidemiological and experimental evidence that EPA and DHA exert protective effects against some common cancers of the breast, colon and perhaps prostate. Veronique Chajès and Philippe Bougnoux in their paper 'Omega–6/Omega–3 Polyunsaturated Fatty Acid Ratio and Cancer' review the experimental and epidemiological evidence, and their own clinical intervention studies, and suggest that the most important aspect of PUFA in the prevention of cancer is the ratio of omega–6 to omega–3 PUFA rather than the absolute amount of either. In Western diets, the omega–6/omega–3 PUFA ratio is 15/1 to 16.7/1. Epidemiological and experimental research indicates that an omega–6/omega–3 PUFA ratio of about 1/1–2/1 has a protective effect against the development and growth of breast and colon cancers. Short-term biomarker studies in human beings suggest that omega–3 PUFA supplementation at a ratio of omega–6 to omega–3 PUFA of about 2.5/1 may protect against colorectal carcinogenesis. Little information is yet available on the role of omega–6 PUFA relative to omega–3 PUFA on prostate cancer, and the findings are controversial.

Leslie Cleland, Michael J. James and Susanna M. Proudman in their paper 'Omega–6/Omega–3 Fatty Acids and Arthritis' discuss the importance of omega–3 fatty acids in reducing pain and inflammation in patients with rheumatoid arthritis and osteoarthritis, as well as improving the outcome in patients with Crohn's disease and IgA nephropathy. They state, 'Because ω6 and ω3 long chain highly unsaturated fatty acids (HUFA) and their polyunsaturated fatty acid (PUFA) metabolic precursors must be acquired from the diet, diet can have an important influence on the likelihood and response to therapy of inflammatory diseases. Therapeutic strategies that reduce ω6 HUFA and increase ω3 HUFA ideally should involve reduced intake of ω6 PUFA in favor of monounsaturates and ω3 PUFA, and increased intake of ω3 HUFA, of which fish oil is a particularly rich source.' There is a strong rationale for reducing symptoms of arthritis based on studies of inhibitory effects of dietary fish oil on production of prostaglandin E_2. Inhibition of thromboxane A_2 (TXA$_2$), TNF-α, and IL-1 production provide a basis for anticipating better long-term outcomes with omega–3-rich diets. Empirically, strong evidence exists for symptomatic benefit in rheumatoid arthritis. A similar rationale exists for benefit in other arthropathies, although there is little evidence upon which to make an evaluation. Data on effects of dietary omega–3 enrichment on long-term outcomes in rheumatoid arthritis are lacking, although improved outcomes in Crohn's disease and IgA nephropathy provide a basis for optimism.

Between 100 and 150 million people globally suffer from asthma with an annual death toll of over 180,000. Asthma has become more prevalent in much of the developed world since the 1960s, with up to 5% of the population typically affected and is the most common chronic condition of childhood with between 20 and 25% of children experiencing wheezing at some point in their life. The most rapid increase is occurring in children under the age of 5 with a 74% increase between 1980 and 1997. The events of asthma include the activation of a cell-surface esterase, calcium influx, and phospholipase activation leading to arachidonic acid release from a parent phospholipid. As a result of these processes, numerous mediators of asthma are produced including preformed molecules that provide an immediate response, new molecules generated as a result of degranulation of mast cells, and granule-associated mediators that act for an extended period of time. Leukotrienes (LT) and prostaglandins generated from released arachidonic acid as a result of degranulation are classified as newly generated mediators and are involved in the pathological changes associated with asthma.

Leukotrienes C_4 and D_4 mediate bronchial smooth-muscle contraction, mucosal edema, and mucus secretion, with LTB_4 promoting cellular infiltration. It is possible to modify the pattern if LT biosynthesis through specific lipid modifications of the diet with extensive research having been conducted over the past 3 decades. Interest in the role of specific lipids and their influence in asthma has focused on the role of the omega–6 and omega–3 PUFA in the potential amelioration of asthma symptoms as these two families of lipids have the potential to significantly alter the course of eicosanoid biosynthesis.

Based on initial observations in populations that consume high levels of omega–3 PUFA and display a low incidence of asthma, many studies have been conducted examining if omega–3 PUFA consumption would be an effective means of ameliorating asthma symptoms. While increased consumption of omega–6 fatty acids does not lead to an improvement in asthma symptoms, elicitation scores or respiratory parameters, the benefits associated with omega–3 PUFA ingestion have been equivocal. Several studies have demonstrated a benefit while others have not. Still others have shown no general benefit in the overall asthmatic response while others demonstrate a beneficial effect in the late asthmatic response. Short-term feeding may not be effective unless the omega–6 PUFA in the diet are accounted for and long-term feeding may be ineffective if omega–3 PUFA are not fed at a substantial enough level. The benefit when achieved is lost if consumption of omega–3 PUFA is not maintained. Further, the preformed long-chain omega–3 PUFA of marine origin appear to be more effective than α-linolenic acid found in vegetable oils.

Many of the chronic conditions – cardiovascular disease, diabetes, cancer, obesity, autoimmune diseases, rheumatoid arthritis, asthma and depression–are associated with increased production of TXA_2, leukotriene B_4 (LTB_4), IL-1β, IL-6, TNF, and CRP. All these factors increase by increases in omega–6 fatty acid intake, and decrease by increases in omega–3 fatty acid intake, either ALA or EPA and DHA. EPA and DHA are more potent, and most studies have been carried out using EPA and DHA.

The optimal range of the ratio of omega–6/omega–3 varies from 1/1 to 4/1 depending on the disease under consideration. Studies show that the background diet, when balanced in omega–6/omega–3, reduces the drug dose. It is therefore essential to decrease the omega–6 intake while increasing the omega–3 in the prevention and management of chronic diseases. Furthermore, the balance of omega–6 and omega–3 fatty acids is very important for homeostasis and normal development. The ratio of omega–6 to omega–3 essential fatty acids is an important determinant of health. In making dietary recommendations, omega–6 and omega–3 PUFA should be distinguished in food labels because they are metabolically and functionally distinct.

This volume should be of interest to a large and varied audience of researchers in academia, industry, and government; cardiologists, geneticists, immunologists, neuroscientists, and cancer specialists; as well as nutritionists, dietitians, food scientists, agriculturists, economists and regulators.

Artemis P. Simopoulos, MD

Simopoulos AP, Cleland LG (eds): Omega–6/Omega–3 Essential Fatty Acid Ratio:
The Scientific Evidence. World Rev Nutr Diet. Basel, Karger, 2003, vol 92, pp 1–22

....

Importance of the Ratio of Omega–6/Omega–3 Essential Fatty Acids: Evolutionary Aspects

A.P. Simopoulos

The Center for Genetics, Nutrition and Health, Washington, D.C., USA

The interaction of genetics and environment, nature, and nurture is the foundation for all health and disease. In the last two decades, using the techniques of molecular biology, it has been shown that genetic factors determine susceptibility to disease and environmental factors determine which genetically susceptible individuals will be affected [1–5]. Nutrition is an environmental factor of major importance. Whereas major changes have taken place in our diet over the past 10,000 years since the beginning of the Agricultural Revolution, our genes have not changed. The spontaneous mutation rate for nuclear DNA is estimated at 0.5% per million years. Therefore, over the past 10,000 years there has been time for very little change in our genes, perhaps 0.005%. In fact, our genes today are very similar to the genes of our ancestors during the Paleolithic period 40,000 years ago, at which time our genetic profile was established [6]. Genetically speaking, humans today live in a nutritional environment that differs from that for which our genetic constitution was selected. Studies on the evolutionary aspects of diet indicate that major changes have taken place in our diet, particularly in the type and amount of essential fatty acids and in the antioxidant content of foods [6–10] (table 1; fig. 1). Using the tools of molecular biology and genetics, research is defining the mechanisms by which genes influence nutrient absorption, metabolism and excretion, taste perception, and degree of satiation; and the mechanisms by which nutrients influence gene expression.

Whereas evolutionary maladaptation leads to reproductive restriction (or differential fertility), the rapid changes in our diet, particularly the last 100 years, are potent promoters of chronic diseases such as atherosclerosis, essential hypertension, obesity, diabetes, and many cancers. In addition to diet,

Table 1. Characteristics of hunter-gatherer and western diet and lifestyles

Characteristic	Hunter-gatherer diet and lifestyle	Western diet and lifestyle
Physical activity level	high	low
Diet		
Energy density	low	high
Energy intake	moderate	high
Protein	high	low-moderate
Animal	high	low-moderate
Vegetable	very low	low-moderate
Carbohydrate	low-moderate (slowly absorbed)	moderate (rapidly absorbed)
Fiber	high	low
Fat	low	high
Animal	low	high
Vegetable	very low	moderate to high
Total long-chain ω6 + ω3	high (2.3 g/day)	low (0.2 g/day)
Ratio ω6/ω3	low (2.4)	high (12.0)
Vitamins, mg/day	*Paleolithic period*	*Current US intake*
Riboflavin	6.49	1.34–2.08
Folate	0.357	0.149–0.205
Thiamin	3.91	1.08–1.75
Ascorbate	604	77–109
Carotene	5.56	2.05–2.57
(Retinol equivalent)	(927)	–
Vitamin A	17.2	7.02–8.48
(Retinol equivalent)	(2,870)	(1,170–429)
Vitamin E	32.8	7–10

Modified from Simopoulos [8].

sedentary lifestyles and exposure to noxious substances interact with genetically controlled biochemical processes leading to chronic disease. This paper reviews the scientific evidence for a balanced intake of omega–6 and omega–3 essential fatty acids (EFA), focusing on the evolutionary aspects of diet, the biological and metabolic functions, and the health implications. Appendix I is a portion of the summary of The Workshop on the Essentiality of and Recommended Dietary Intakes (RDIs) for Omega–6 and Omega–3 Fatty Acids, held at the National Institutes of Health (NIH) in Bethesda, Md., USA, April 7–9, 1999, which provides recommendations for adequate intakes (AI) of essential fatty acids (EFA) for adults and infants [11].

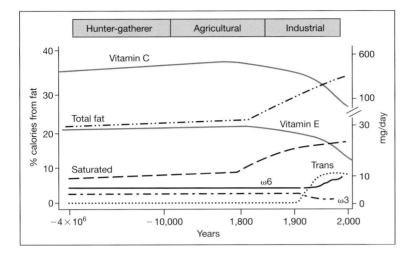

Fig. 1. Hypothetical scheme of fat, fatty acid (ω6, ω3, trans and total) intake (as percent of calories from fat) and intake of vitamins E and C (mg/d). Data were extrapolated from cross-sectional analyses of contemporary hunter-gatherer populations and from longitudinal observations and their putative changes during the preceding 100 years [8].

Evolutionary Aspects of Diet with Emphasis on Omega–6 and Omega–3 Essential Fatty Acids

The foods that were commonly available to pre-agricultural humans (lean meat, fish, green leafy vegetables, fruits, nuts, berries and honey) were the foods that shaped modern humans' genetic nutritional requirements. Cereal grains as a staple food are a relatively recent addition to the human diet and represent a dramatic departure from those foods to which we are genetically programmed and adapted [12–14]. Cereals did not become a part of our food supply till only very recently – 10,000 years ago – with the advent of the Agricultural Revolution. Prior to the Agricultural Revolution humans ate an enormous variety of wild plants, whereas today about 17% of plant species provide 90% of the world's food supply, with the greatest percentage contributed by cereal grains [12–14]. Three cereals (wheat, maize, and rice) together account for 75% of the world's grain production. Human beings have become entirely dependent upon cereal grains for the greater portion of their food supply. The nutritional implications of such a high grain consumption upon human health are enormous. Cereal grains are high in carbohydrates and omega–6 fatty acids, but low in omega–3 fatty acids and in antioxidants, particularly in comparison to green leafy vegetables. Recent studies show that low-fat/high-carbohydrate diets increase insulin resistance and hyperinsulinemia, conditions that increase the risk for coronary heart disease, hypertension, diabetes and obesity [15–18]. And yet, for the 99.9% of mankind's presence on this planet, humans rarely or never consumed cereal grains. It is only since the last 10,000 years that humans consume cereals. Up to that time, humans were non-cereal-eating hunter-gatherers since the emergence of *Homo erectus* 1.7 million years ago. There is no evolutionary precedent in our species for grass seed consumption [6, 12]. Therefore, we had little time (<500 generations) since the beginning of the Agricultural Revolution 10,000 years ago to adapt to a food type which now represents humanity's major source of both calories and protein. A number of anthropological, nutritional and genetic studies indicate that human's overall diet, including energy intake and energy expenditure, has changed over the past 10,000 years with major changes occurring during the past 150 years in the type and amount of fat and in vitamins C and E intake [6, 8, 13, 19–24] (tables 1, 2; fig. 1).

Eaton and Konner [6] have estimated higher intakes for protein, calcium, potassium and ascorbic acid and lower sodium intakes for the diet of the late Paleolithic period than the current US and Western diets. Most of our food is calorically concentrated in comparison with the wild game and uncultivated fruits and vegetables of the Paleolithic diet. Paleolithic man consumed fewer calories and drank water, whereas today most thirst-quenching drinks contain calories. Today industrialized societies are characterized by (1) an increase in energy intake and decrease in energy expenditure; (2) an increase in saturated fat, omega–6 fatty acids and *trans* fatty acids, and a decrease in omega–3 fatty acid intake; (3) a decrease in complex carbohydrates and fiber; (4) an increase in cereal grains and a decrease in fruits and vegetables, and (5) a decrease in protein, antioxidants and calcium intake [6, 8, 19–21, 23] (tables 1–3). The increase in *trans* fatty acids is detrimental to health, as shown in table 4 [25]. In addition, *trans* fatty acids interfere with the desaturation and elongation of both omega–6 and omega–3 fatty acids, thus further decreasing the amount of arachidonic acid, eicosapentaenoic acid and docosahexaenoic acid availability for human metabolism [26].

Essential Fatty Acids and the Omega–6/Omega–3 Balance

Large-Scale Production of Vegetable Oils
The increased consumption of omega–6 fatty acids in the last 100 years is due to the development of technology at the turn of the century that marked the beginning of the modern vegetable oil industry, and to modern agriculture with the emphasis on grain feeds for domestic livestock (grains are rich in

Table 2. Estimated omega–6 and omega–3 fatty acid intake in the late Paleolithic period (g/day)[a,b]

Plants	
LA	4.28
ALA	11.40
Animals	
LA	4.56
ALA	1.21
Total	
LA	8.84
ALA	12.60
Animal	
AA (ω6)	1.81
EPA (ω3)	0.39
DTA (ω6)	0.12
DPA (ω3)	0.42
DHA (ω3)	0.27
Ratios of ω6/ω3	
LA/ALA	0.70
AA + DTA/EPA + DPA + DHA	1.79
Total ω6/ω3	0.79[b]

LA = Linoleic acid; ALA = alpha-linolenic acid; AA = arachidonic acid; EPA = eicosapentaenoic acid; DTA = docosatetraenoic acid; DPA = docosapentaenoic acid; DHA = docosahexaenoic acid.

[a]Data from Eaton et al. [20].

[b]Assuming an energy intake of 35:65 of animal:plant sources.

omega–6 fatty acids) [27]. The invention of the continuous screw press, named Expeller® by V.D. Anderson, and the steam-vacuum deodorization process by D. Wesson made possible the industrial production of cottonseed oil and other vegetable oils for cooking [27]. Solvent extraction of oilseeds came into increased use after World War I and the large-scale production of vegetable oils became more efficient and more economic. Subsequently, hydrogenation was applied to oils to solidify them. The partial selective hydrogenation of soybean oil reduced the alpha-linolenic acid (ALA) content of the oil while leaving a high concentration of linoleic acid (LA). ALA content was reduced because ALA in soybean oil caused many organoleptic problems. It is now well known that the hydrogenation process and particularly the formation of *trans* fatty acids has led to increases in serum cholesterol concentrations

Table 3. Late Paleolithic and currently recommended nutrient composition for Americans

	Late Paleolithic	Current recommendations
Total dietary energy, %		
Protein	33	12
Carbohydrate	46	58
Fat	21	30
Alcohol	~0	–
P/S ratio	1.41	1.00
Cholesterol, mg	520	300
Fiber, g	100–150	30–60
Sodium, mg	690	1,100–3,300
Calcium, mg	1,500–2,000	800–1,600
Ascorbic acid, mg	440	60

Modified from Eaton et al. [20]. P/S = Polyunsaturated to saturated fat.

Table 4. Ethnic differences in fatty acid concentrations in thrombocyte phospholipids and percentage of all deaths from cardiovascular disease[1]

	Europe and United States, %	Japan, %	Greenland Eskimos, %
Arachidonic acid ($20:4\omega6$)	26	21	8.3
Eicosapentaenoic acid ($20:5\omega3$)	0.5	1.6	8.0
Ratio of $\omega6/\omega3$	50	12	1
Mortality from cardiovascular disease	45	12	7

[1]Modified from Weber [48].

whereas LA in its regular state in oil is associated with a reduced serum cholesterol concentration [28, 29]. The effects of *trans* fatty acids on health have been reviewed extensively elsewhere [26, 30].

Since the 1950s, research on the effects of omega–6 PUFAs in lowering serum cholesterol concentrations has dominated the research support on the role of PUFAs in lipid metabolism. Although a number of investigators contributed extensively, the paper by Ahrens et al. [31] in 1954 and subsequent work by Keys et al. [32] firmly established the omega–6 fatty acids as the important fatty acid in the field of cardiovascular disease. The availability of methods for the production of vegetable oils and their use in lowering serum cholesterol concentration led to an increase in both the fat content of the diet and the greater increase in vegetable oils rich in omega–6 fatty acids.

Agribusiness and Modern Agriculture

Agribusiness contributed further to the decrease in omega–3 fatty acids in animal carcasses. Wild animals and birds who feed on wild plants are very lean with a carcass fat content of only 3.9% [33] and contain about five times more PUFAs per gram than is found in domestic livestock [20, 34]. Most importantly, 4% of the fat of wild animals contains eicosapentaenoic acid (EPA). Domestic beef contains very small or undetectable amounts of ALA because cattle are fed grains rich in omega–6 fatty acids and poor in omega–3 fatty acids [35] whereas deer that forage on ferns and mosses contain more omega–3 fatty acids (ALA) in their meat.

Modern agriculture with its emphasis on production has decreased the omega–3 fatty acid content in many foods. In addition to animal meats mentioned above [20, 33–35], green leafy vegetables [36–41], eggs [42, 43], and even fish [44] contain less omega–3 fatty acids than those in the wild. Foods from edible wild plants contain a good balance of omega–6 and omega–3 fatty acids. Purslane, an edible wild plant, has 8 times more alpha-linolenic acid than the cultivated plants, such as spinach, red leaf lettuce or mustard greens [36–38]. Modern aquaculture produces fish that contain less omega–3 fatty acids than do fish grown naturally in the ocean, rivers and lakes [44]. The fatty acid composition of egg yolk from free-ranging chickens in the Ampelistra farm in Greece has an omega–6/omega–3 ratio of 1.3 whereas the USDA egg has a ratio of 19.9 [42, 43]. By enriching the chicken feed with fishmeal or flax, the ratio of omega–6/omega–3 decreased to 6.6 and 1.6, respectively [42, 43]. Similarly, milk and cheese from animals that graze contain AA, EPA and DHA, whereas milk and cheese from grain-fed animals do not [23].

Imbalance of Omega–6/Omega–3

It is evident that food technology and agribusiness provided the economic stimulus that dominated the changes in the food supply [45, 46]. From per capita quantities of foods available for consumption in the US national food supply in 1985, the amount of EPA is reported to be about 50 mg per capita/day and the amount of DHA is 80 mg per capita/day. The two main sources are fish and poultry [47]. It has been estimated that the present Western diet is 'deficient' in omega–3 fatty acids with a ratio of omega–6 to omega–3 of 15–20/1, instead of 1/1 as is the case with wild animals and presumably human beings [6–10, 20, 33–35].

Table 5. Omega–6:omega–3 ratios in various populations

Population	ω6/ω3	Reference
Paleolithic	0.79	[20]
Greece prior to 1960	1.00–2.00	[23]
Current Japan	4.00	[51]
Current India, rural	5–6.1	[52]
Current United Kingdom and northern Europe	15.00	[53]
Current United States	16.74	[20]
Current India, urban	38–50	[52]

Before the 1940s cod-liver oil was ingested mainly by children as a source of vitamin A and D with the usual dose being a teaspoon. Once these vitamins were synthesized, consumption of cod-liver oil was drastically decreased, contributing further to the decrease of EPA and DHA intake. Table 4 shows ethnic differences in fatty acid concentrations in thrombocyte phospholipids, the ratios of omega–6/omega–3 fatty acids, and percentage of all deaths from cardiovascular disease [48].

Thus, an absolute and relative change of omega–6/omega–3 in the food supply of Western societies has occurred over the last 100 years. A balance existed between omega–6 and omega–3 for millions of years during the long evolutionary history of the genus *Homo*, and genetic changes occurred partly in response to these dietary influences. During evolution, omega–3 fatty acids were found in all foods consumed: meat, wild plants, eggs, fish, nuts and berries. Recent studies by Cordain et al. [49] on wild animals confirm the original observations of Crawford and Sinclair et al. [34, 50]. However, rapid dietary changes over short periods of time as have occurred over the past 100–150 years is a totally new phenomenon in human evolution (table 5) [20, 23, 51–53].

Biological Effects and Metabolic Functions of Omega–6 and Omega–3 Fatty Acids

Mammalian cells cannot convert omega–6 to omega–3 fatty acids because they lack the converting enzyme, omega–3 desaturase. LA and ALA and their long-chain derivatives are important components of animal and plant cell membranes. These two classes of EFA are not interconvertible, are metabolically and functionally distinct, and often have important opposing physiological functions. The balance of EFA is important for good health and normal development.

Table 6. Effects of ingestion of EPA and DHA from fish or fish oil

- Decreased production of prostaglandin E_2 (PGE_2) metabolites
- A decrease in thromboxane A_2, a potent platelet aggregator and vasoconstrictor
- A decrease in leukotriene B_4 formation, an inducer of inflammation, and a powerful inducer of leukocyte chemotaxis and adherence
- An increase in thromboxane A_3, a weak platelet aggregator and weak vasoconstrictor
- An increase in prostacyclin PGI_3, leading to an overall increase in total prostacyclin by increasing PGI_3 without a decrease in PGI_2, both PGI_2 and PGI_3 are active vasodilators and inhibitors of platelet aggregation
- An increase in leukotriene B_5, a weak inducer of inflammation and a weak chemotactic agent

When humans ingest fish or fish oil, the EPA and DHA from the diet partially replace the omega–6 fatty acids, especially AA, in the membranes of probably all cells, but especially in the membranes of platelets, erythrocytes, neutrophils, monocytes, and liver cells [reviewed in ref. 7]. Whereas cellular proteins are genetically determined, the PUFA composition of cell membranes is to a great extent dependent on the dietary intake. AA and EPA are the parent compounds for eicosanoid production (table 6; fig. 2).

Because of the increased amounts of omega–6 fatty acids in the Western diet, the eicosanoid metabolic products from AA, specifically prostaglandins, thromboxanes, leukotrienes, hydroxy fatty acids, and lipoxins, are formed in larger quantities than those formed from omega–3 fatty acids, specifically EPA. The eicosanoids from AA are biologically active in very small quantities and, if they are formed in large amounts, they contribute to the formation of thrombus and atheromas; to allergic and inflammatory disorders, particularly in suscepti-ble people; and to proliferation of cells. Thus, a diet rich in omega–6 fatty acids shifts the physiological state to one that is prothrombotic and proaggregatory, with increases in blood viscosity, vasospasm, and vasoconstriction and decreases in bleeding time. Bleeding time is decreased in groups of patients with hyper-cholesterolemia [54], hyperlipoproteinemia [55], myocardial infarction, other forms of atherosclerotic disease, and diabetes (obesity and hypertrigly-ceridemia). Bleeding time is longer in women than in men and longer in young than in old people. There are ethnic differences in bleeding time that appear to be related to diet. Table 4 shows that the higher the ratio of omega–6/omega–3 fatty acids in platelet phospholipids, the higher the death rate from cardio-vascular disease [7, 48].

The antithrombotic aspects and the effects of different doses of fish oil on the prolongation of bleeding time were investigated by Saynor et al. [56]. A dose of 1.8 g/day EPA did not result in any prolongation in bleeding time, but at 4 g/day

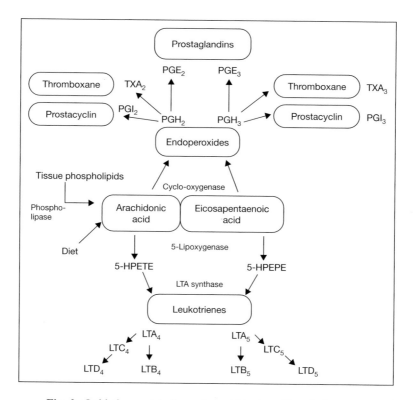

Fig. 2. Oxidative metabolism of arachidonic acid and eicosapentaenoic acid by the cyclooxygenase and 5-lipoxygenase pathways. 5-HPETE denotes 5-hydroperoxyeicosatetra-noic acid and 5-HPEPE denotes 5-hydroxyeicosapentaenoic acid.

the bleeding time increased and the platelet count decreased without any adverse effects. In human studies there has never been a case of clinical bleeding, even in patients undergoing angioplasty while they were on fish oil supplements [57].

There is substantial agreement that ingestion of fish or fish oils has the following effects: platelet aggregation to epinephrine and collagen is inhibited, thromboxane A_2 production is decreased, whole blood viscosity is reduced, and erythrocyte membrane fluidity is increased [58–61] (table 7). Fish oil ingestion increases the concentration of plasminogen activator and decreases the concentration of plasminogen activator inhibitor 1 (PAI-1) [62]. In vitro studies have demonstrated that PAI-1 is synthesized and secreted in hepatic cells in response to insulin, and population studies indicate a strong correlation between insulinemia and PAI-1 levels. In patients with types IIb and IV hyperlipoproteinemia and in another double-blind clinical trial involving 64 men aged 35–40 years, ingestion of omega–3 fatty acids decreased the fibrinogen concentration [63].

Table 7. Effects of omega–3 fatty acids on factors involved in the pathophysiology of inflammation

Factor	Function	Effect of ω3 fatty acid
Arachidonic acid	eicosanoid precursor; aggregates platelets; stimulates white blood cells	↓
Thromboxane	platelet aggregation; vasoconstriction; increase of intracellular Ca^{2++}	↓
Prostacyclin ($PGI_{2/3}$)	prevent platelet aggregation; vasodilation; increase cAMP	↑
Leukotriene (LTB_4)	neutrophil chemoattractant; increase of intracellular Ca^{2++}	↓
Fibrinogen	a member of the acute phase response; and a blood clotting factor	↓
Tissue plasminogen activator	increase endogenous fibrinolysis	↑
Platelet-activating factor (PAF)	activates platelets and white blood cells	↓
Platelet-derived growth factor (PDGF)	chemoattractant and mitogen for smooth muscles and macrophages	↓
Oxygen free radicals	cellular damage; enhance LDL uptake via scavenger pathway; stimulate arachidonic acid metabolism	↓
Lipid hydroperoxides	stimulate eicosanoid formation	↓
Interleukin-1 and tumor necrosis factor	stimulate neutrophil O_2 free radical formation; stimulate lymphocyte proliferation; stimulate PAF; express intercellular adhesion molecule-1 on endothelial cells; inhibit plasminogen activator, thus, procoagulants	↓
Interleukin-6	stimulates the synthesis of all acute phase proteins involved in the inflammatory response: C-reative protein; serum amyloid A; fibrinogen; α_1-chymotrypsin; and haptoglobin	↓

Adapted and modified from Weber and Leaf [61].

Two other studies did not show a decrease in fibrinogen, but in one a small dose of cod-liver oil was used [64] and in the other the study consisted of normal volunteers and was of short duration. A recent study noted that fish and fish oil increase fibrinolytic activity, indicating that 200 g/day of lean fish or 2 g of omega–3 EPA and DHA improve certain hematologic parameters implicated in the etiology of cardiovascular disease [65].

Ingestion of omega–3 fatty acids not only increases the production of PGI_3, but also of PGI_2 in tissue fragments from the atrium, aorta, and saphenous vein obtained at surgery in patients who received fish oil 2 weeks prior to surgery [66]. Omega–3 fatty acids inhibit the production of platelet-derived growth factor (PDGF) in bovine endothelial cells [67]. PDGF is a chemoattractant for smooth muscle cells and a powerful mitogen. Thus, the reduction in its production by endothelial cells, monocytes/macrophages, and platelets could inhibit both the migration and proliferation of smooth muscle cells, monocytes/macrophages, and fibroblasts in the arterial wall. Insulin increases the growth of smooth muscle cells, leading to increased risk for the development of atherosclerosis. Omega–3 fatty acids increase endothelium-derived relaxing factor (EDRF) [68]. EDRF (nitric oxide) facilitates relaxation in large arteries and vessels. In the presence of EPA, endothelial cells in culture increase the release of relaxing factors, indicating a direct effect of omega–3 fatty acids on the cells.

Many experimental studies have provided evidence that incorporation of alternative fatty acids into tissues may modify inflammatory and immune reactions and that omega–3 fatty acids in particular are potent therapeutic agents for inflammatory diseases. Supplementing the diet with omega–3 fatty acids (3.2 g EPA and 2.2 g DHA) in normal subjects increased the EPA content in neutrophils and monocytes more than sevenfold without changing the quantities of AA and DHA. The anti-inflammatory effects of fish oils are partly mediated by inhibiting the 5-lipoxygenase pathway in neutrophils and monocytes and inhibiting the leukotriene B_4 (LTB_4)-mediated function of LTB_5 (fig. 2) [69, 70]. Studies show that omega–3 fatty acids influence interleukin metabolism by decreasing IL-1β and IL-6 [71–74]. Inflammation plays an important role in both the initiation of atherosclerosis and the development of atherothrombotic events [75]. An early step in the atherosclerotic process is the adhesion of monocytes to endothelial cells. Adhesion is mediated by leukocyte and vascular cell adhesion molecules (CAMs) such as selectins, integrins, vascular cell adhesion molecule 1 (VCAM-1), and intercellular adhesion molecule 1 (ICAM-1) [76]. The expression of E-selectin, ICAM-1 and VCAM-1, which is relatively low in normal vascular cells, is upregulated in the presence of various stimuli, including cytokines and oxidants. This increased expression promotes the adhesion of monocytes to the vessel wall. The monocytes subsequently migrate across the endothelium into the vascular intima, where they accumulate to form the initial lesions of atherosclerosis. Atherosclerotic plaques have been shown to have increased CAM expression in animal models and human studies [77–80]. A balance between the omega–6 and omega–3 fatty acids is a more physiologic state in terms of gene expression [81], eicosanoid metabolism and cytokine production.

Further support for the need to balance the omega–6/omega–3 EFA comes from the studies of Ge et al. [82] and Kang et al. [83]. The study by Ge et al. [82] clearly shows the ability of both normal rat cardiomyocytes and human breast cancer cells in culture to form all the omega–3s from omega–6 fatty acids when fed the cDNA encoding omega–3 fatty acid desaturase obtained from the roundworm *Caenorhabitis elegans*. The omega–3 desaturase efficiently and quickly converted the omega–6 fatty acids that were fed to the cardiomyocytes in culture to the corresponding omega–3 fatty acids. Thus, omega–6 LA was converted to omega–3 ALA and AA was converted to EPA, so that at equilibrium, the ratio of omega–6 to omega–3 PUFA was close to 1/1 [83]. Further studies demonstrated that the cancer cells expressing the omega–3 desaturase underwent apoptotic death whereas the control cancer cells with a high omega–6/omega–3 ratio continued to proliferate [82].

Clinical Intervention Studies and the Omega–6/Omega–3 EFA Balance

This volume includes papers on clinical intervention studies that emphasize the importance of the omega–6/omega–3 ratio in coronary heart disease [52, 84–85], brain function [86], cancer [87] and arthritis[88].

Psychologic stress in humans induces the production of proinflammatory cytokines such as interferon-γa (IFNγ), TNFα, IL-6 and IL-10. An imbalance of omega–6 and omega–3 PUFA in the peripheral blood causes an overproduction of proinflammatory cytokines. There is evidence that changes in fatty acid composition are involved in the pathophysiology of major depression. Changes in serotonin (5-HT) receptor number and function caused by changes in PUFA provide the theoretical rationale connecting fatty acids with the current receptor and neurotransmitter theories of depression [89–91]. The increased C20:4ω6/C20:5ω3 ratio and the imbalance in the omega–6/omega–3 PUFA ratio in major depression may be related to the increased production of proinflammatory cytokines and eicosanoids in that illness [89]. There are a number of studies evaluating the therapeutic effect of EPA and DHA in major depression. Stoll and colleagues have shown that EPA and DHA prolong remission, that is, reduce the risk of relapse in patients with bipolar disorder [92, 93].

The clinical studies in patients with cardiovascular disease, arthritis, asthma, cancer, and mental illness clearly indicate the need to balance the omega–6/omega–3 fatty acid intake for prevention and during treatment. The scientific evidence is strong for decreasing the omega–6 and increasing the omega–3 intake to improve health throughout the life cycle. The scientific basis for the development of a public policy to develop dietary recommendations for essential fatty acids, including a balanced omega–6/omega–3 ratio is robust [94]. What is needed is a scientific consensus, education of professionals and the public, the establishment of an agency on nutrition and food policy at the national level, and willingness of governments to institute changes. Education of the public is essential to demand changes in the food supply.

Conclusions

- Human beings evolved on a diet in which the ratio of omega–6/omega–3 EFA was about 1, whereas in the Western diets the ratio is 15/1 to 16.7/1. Evidence comes from studies on the evolutionary aspects of diet, modern day hunter-gatherers, and traditional diets. Agribusiness and modern agriculture have led to decreases in omega–3 fatty acids and increases in omega–6 fatty acids. Such practices have led to excessive amounts of omega–6 fatty acids, upsetting the balance that was characteristic during evolution when our genes were programmed to respond to diet and other aspects of the environment.
- LA and ALA are not interconvertible and compete for the rate-limiting delta–6-desaturase in the synthesis of long-chain PUFA.
- AA (omega–6) and EPA (omega–3) are the parent compounds for the production of eicosanoids. Eicosanoids from AA have opposing properties from those of EPA. An increase in the dietary intake of omega–6 EFA changes the physiological state to a prothrombotic, proconstrictive, and proinflammatory.
- Many of the chronic conditions – cardiovascular disease, diabetes, cancer, obesity, autoimmune diseases, rheumatoid arthritis, asthma and depression – are associated with increased production of thromboxane A_2 (TXA$_2$), leukotriene B_4 (LTB$_4$), IL-1β, IL-6, tumor necrosis factor (TNF), and C-reactive protein. All these factors increase by increases in omega–6 fatty acid intake and decrease by increases in omega–3 fatty acid intake, either ALA or EPA and DHA. EPA and DHA are more potent, and most studies have been carried out using EPA and DHA.
- The optimal dose or ratio of omega–6/omega–3 varies from 1/1 to 4/1 depending on the disease under consideration. Since many of the chronic

diseases prevalent in Western cultures are multigenic and multifactorial, it is not surprising that the dose or the ratio differs.

- Studies show that the background diet when balanced in omega–6/omega–3 decreases the drug dose. It is therefore essential to decrease the omega–6 intake while increasing the omega–3 in the prevention and management of chronic disease. Furthermore, the balance of omega–6 and omega–3 fatty acids is very important for homeostasis and normal development. The ratio of omega–6 to omega–3 EFA is an important determinant of health. Therefore, appropriate amounts of dietary omega–6 and omega–3 fatty acids at a ratio of about 1–2/1 consistent with the recommended AI found in tables 1 and 2 of Appendix I, need to be considered in making dietary recommendations, and these two classes of PUFA should be distinguished in food labels because they are metabolically and functionally distinct.

References

1   Simopoulos AP, Childs B (eds): Genetic Variation and Nutrition. Wld Rev Nutr Diet. Basel, Karger, 1990, vol 63.
2   Simopoulos AP, Herbert V, Jacobson B: The Healing Diet: How to Reduce Your Risks and Live a Longer and Healthier Life If You Have a Family History of Cancer, Heart Disease, Hypertension, Diabetes, Alcoholism, Obesity, Food Allergies. New York, Macmillan, 1995.
3   Simopoulos AP, Nestel PJ (eds): Genetic Variation and Dietary Response. World Rev Nutr Diet. Basel, Karger, 1997, vol 80.
4   Simopoulos AP, Pavlou KN (eds): Nutrition and Fitness. 1. Diet, Genes, Physical Activity and Health. Proceedings of the Fourth International Conference on Nutrition and Fitness, Ancient Olympia, Greece, May 25–29, 2000. World Rev Nutr Diet. Basel, Karger, 2001, vol 89.
5   Simopoulos AP: Genetic variation and dietary response: Nutrigenetics/nutrigenomics. Asia Pacific J Clin Nutr 2002;11(S6):S117–S128.
6   Eaton SB, Konner M: Paleolithic nutrition: A consideration of its nature and current implications. N Engl J Med 1985;312:283–289.
7   Simopoulos AP: Omega–3 fatty acids in health and disease and in growth and development. Am J Clin Nutr 1991;54:438–463.
8   Simopoulos AP: Genetic variation and evolutionary aspects of diet; in Papas A (ed): Antioxidants in Nutrition and Health. Boca Raton, CRC Press, 1999, pp 65–88.
9   Simopoulos AP: Evolutionary aspects of omega–3 fatty acids in the food supply. Prostaglandins Leukotrienes Essential Fatty Acids. 1999;60:421–429.
10 Simopoulos AP: New products from the agri-food industry: The return of n–3 fatty acids into the food supply. Lipids 1999;34(suppl):S297–S301.
11 Simopoulos AP, Leaf A, Salem N Jr: Essentiality of and recommended dietary intakes for omega–6 and omega–3 fatty acids. Ann Nutr Metab 1999;43:127–130.
12 Cordain L: Cereal grains: Humanity's double-edged sword; in Simopoulos AP (ed): Evolutionary Aspects of Nutrition and Health. Diet, Exercise, Genetics and Chronic Disease. World Rev Nutr Diet. Basel, Karger, 1999, vol 84, pp19–73.
13 Simopoulos AP (ed): Plants in Human Nutrition. World Rev Nutr Diet. Basel, Karger, 1995, vol 77.
14 Simopoulos AP (ed): Evolutionary Aspects of Nutrition and Health. Diet, Exercise, Genetics and Chronic Disease. World Rev Nutr Diet. Basel, Karger, 1999, vol 84.

15   Fanaian M, Szilasi J, Storlien L, Calvert GD: The effect of modified fat diet on insulin resistance and metabolic parameters in type II diabetes. Diabetologia 1996;39(suppl 1):A7.

16   Simopoulos AP: Is insulin resistance influenced by dietary linoleic acid and trans fatty acids? Free Rad Biol Med 1994;17:367–372.

17   Simopoulos AP: Fatty acid composition of skeletal muscle membrane phospholipids, insulin resistance and obesity. Nutr Today 1994;2:12–16.

18   Simopoulos AP, Robinson J: The Omega Diet. The Lifesaving Nutritional Program Based on the Diet of the Island of Crete. New York, Harper Collins, 1999.

19   Eaton SB, Konner M, Shostak M: Stone agers in the fast lane: Chronic degenerative diseases in evolutionary perspective. Am J Med 1988;84:739–749.

20   Eaton SB, Eaton SB III, Sinclair AJ, Cordain L, Mann NJ: Dietary intake of long-chain poly-unsaturated fatty acids during the Paleolithic; in Simopoulos AP (ed): The Return of ω3 Fatty Acids into the Food Supply. I. Land-Based Animal Food Products and Their Health Effects. World Rev Nutr Diet. Basel, Karger, 1998, vol 83, pp 12–23.

21   Leaf A, Weber PC: A new era for science in nutrition. Am J Clin Nutr 1987;45:1048–1053.

22   Simopoulos AP: The Mediterranean diet: Greek column rather than an Egyptian pyramid. Nutr Today 1995;30:54–61.

23   Simopoulos AP: Overview of evolutionary aspects of ω3 fatty acids in the diet; in Simopoulos AP (ed): The Return of ω3 Fatty Acids into the Food Supply. I. Land-Based Animal Food Products and Their Health Effects. World Rev Nutr Diet. Basel, Karger, 1998, vol 83, pp 1–11.

24   Simopoulos AP: Evolutionary aspects of diet and essential fatty acids. World Rev Nutr Diet. Basel, Karger, 2001, vol 88, pp 18–27.

25   Simopoulos AP: Evolutionary aspects of diet: Fatty acids, insulin resistance and obesity; in VanItallie TB, Simopoulos AP (senior eds): Obesity: New Directions in Assessment and Management. Philadelphia, Charles Press, 1995, pp 241–261.

26   Simopoulos AP: Trans fatty acids; in Spiller GA (ed): Handbook of Lipids in Human Nutrition. Boca Raton, CRC Press, 1995, pp 91–99.

27   Kirshenbauer HG: Fats and Oils, ed 2. New York, Reinhold, 1960.

28   Emken EA: Nutrition and biochemistry of trans and positional fatty acid isomers in hydrogenated oils. Ann Rev Nutr 1984;4:339–376.

29   Troisi R, Willett WC, Weiss ST: Trans-fatty acid intake in relation to serum lipid concentrations in adult men. Am J Clin Nutr 1992;56:1019–1024.

30   Simopoulos AP: Omega–6/omega–3 fatty acid ratio and trans fatty acids in non-insulin dependent diabetes mellitus: Lipids and syndromes of insulin resistance. Ann NY Acad Sci 1997;827:327–338.

31   Ahrens EH, Blankenhorn DH, Tsaltas TT: Effect on human serum lipids of substituting plant for animal fat in the diet. Proc Soc Exp Biol Med 1954;86:872–878.

32   Keys A, Anderson JT, Grande F: Serum cholesterol response to dietary fat. Lancet 1957;i:787.

33   Ledger HP: Body composition as a basis for a comparative study of some East African animals. Symp Zool Soc Lond 1968;21:289–310.

34   Crawford MA: Fatty acid ratios in free-living and domestic animals. Lancet 1968;i:1329–1333.

35   Crawford MA, Gale MM, Woodford MH: Linoleic acid and linolenic acid elongation products in muscle tissue of *Syncerus caffer* and other ruminant species. Biochem J 1969;115:25–27.

36   Simopoulos AP, Norman HA, Gillaspy JE, Duke JA: Common purslane: A source of omega–3 fatty acids and antioxidants. J Am Coll Nutr 1992;11:374–382.

37   Simopoulos AP, Norman HA, Gillaspy JE: Purslane in human nutrition and its potential for world agriculture; in Simopoulos AP (ed): Plants in Human Nutrition. World Rev Nutr Diet. Basel, Karger, 1995, vol 77, pp 47–74.

38   Simopoulos AP, Salem N Jr: Purslane: A terrestrial source of omega–3 fatty acids. N Engl J Med 1986;315:833.

39   Simopoulos AP, Gopalan C (eds): Plants in Human Health and Nutrition Policy. World Rev Nutr Diet. Basel, Karger, 2003, vol 91.

40   Zeghichi S, Kallithrka S, Simopoulos AP, Kypriotakis Z: Nutritional composition of selected wild plants in the diet of Crete; in Simopoulos AP, Gopalan C (eds): Plants in Human Health and Nutrition Policy. World Rev Nutr Diet. Basel, Karger, 2003, vol 91, pp 22–40.

41   Simopoulos AP: Omega–3 fatty acids in wild plants, seeds and nuts. Asian Pacific J Clin Nutr 2002;11(S6):S163–S173.
42   Simopoulos AP, Salem N Jr: n-3 fatty acids in eggs from range-fed Greek chickens. N Engl J Med 1989;321:1412.
43   Simopoulos AP, Salem N Jr: Egg yolk as a source of long-chain polyunsaturated fatty acids in infant feeding. Am J Clin Nutr 1992;55:411–414.
44   van Vliet T, Katan MB: Lower ratio of n-3 to n-6 fatty acids in cultured than in wild fish. Am J Clin Nutr 1990;51:1–2.
45   Hunter JE: Omega–3 fatty acids from vegetable oils; in Galli C, Simopoulos AP (eds): Biological Effects and Nutritional Essentiality. Series A: Life Sciences. New York, Plenum Press, 1989, vol 171, pp 43–55.
46   Litin L, Sacks F: Trans-fatty-acid content of common foods. N Engl J Med 1993;329:1969–1970.
47   Raper NR, Cronin FJ, Exler J: Omega–3 fatty acid content of the US food supply. J Am College Nutr 1992;11:304.
48   Weber PC: Are we what we eat? Fatty acids in nutrition and in cell membranes: Cell functions and disorders induced by dietary conditions. Svanoybukt, Svanoy Foundation, 1989, report No 4, pp 9–18.
49   Cordain L, Martin C, Florant G, Watkins BA: The fatty acid composition of muscle, brain, marrow and adipose tissue in elk: Evolutionary implications for human dietary requirements; in Simopoulos AP (ed): The Return of ω3 Fatty Acids into the Food Supply. I. Land-Based Animal Food Products and Their Health Effects. World Rev Nutr Diet. Basel, Karger, 1998, vol 83, pp 225.
50   Sinclair AJ, Slattery WJ, O'Dea K: The analysis of polyunsaturated fatty acids in meat by capillary gas-liquid chromotography. J Food Sci Agric 1982;33:771–776.
51   Sugano M, Hirahara F: Polyunsaturated fatty acids in the food chain in Japan. Am J Clin Nutr 2000;71(suppl):189S–196S.
52   Pella D, Dubnov G, Singh RB, Sharma R, Berry EM, Manor O: Effects of an Indo-Mediterranean diet on the omega–6/omega–3 ratio in patients at high risk of coronary artery disease: The Indian paradox. World Rev Nutr Diet. Basel, Karger, 2003, vol 92, pp 74–80.
53   Sanders TAB: Polyunsaturated fatty acids in the food chain in Europe. Am J Clin Nutr 2000;71(suppl):S176–S178.
54   Brox JH, Killie JE, Osterud B, Holme S, Nordoy A: Effects of cod liver oil on platelets and coagulation in familial hypercholesterolemia (type IIa). Acta Med Scand 1983;213:137–144.
55   Joist JH, Baker RK, Schonfeld G: Increased in vivo and in vitro platelet function in type II- and type IV-hyperlipoproteinemia. Thromb Res 1979;15:95–108.
56   Saynor R, Verel D, Gillott T: The long term effect of dietary supplementation with fish lipid concentrate on serum lipids, bleeding time, platelets and angina. Atherosclerosis 1984;50:3–10.
57   Dehmer GJ, Pompa JJ, Van den Berg EK, et al: Reduction in the rate of early restenosis after coronary angioplasty by a diet supplemented with n-3 fatty acids. N Engl J Med 1988;319:733–740.
58   Bottiger LE, Dyerberg J, Nordoy A (eds): n-3 fish oils in clinical medicine. J Intern Med 1989;225(suppl):1–238.
59   Cartwright IJ, Pockley AG, Galloway JH, et al: The effects of dietary ω-3 polyunsaturated fatty acids on erythrocyte membrane phospholipids, erythrocyte deformability, and blood viscosity in healthy volunteers. Atherosclerosis 1985;55:267–281.
60   Lewis RA, Lee TH, Austen KF: Effects of omega–3 fatty acids on the generation of products of the 5-lipoxygenase pathway; in Simopoulos AP, Kifer RR, Martin RE (eds): Health Effects of Polyunsaturated Fatty Acids in Seafoods. Orlando, Academic Press, 1986, pp 227–238.
61   Weber PC, Leaf A: Cardiovascular effects of ω3 fatty acids: Atherosclerotic risk factor modification by ω3 fatty acids; in Simopoulos AP, Kifer RR, Martin RE (eds): Health Effects of ω3 Polyunsaturated Fatty Acids in Seafoods. World Rev Nutr Diet. Basel, Karger, 1991, vol 66, pp 218–232.
62   Barcelli UO, Glass-Greenwalt P, Pollak VE: Enhancing effect of dietary supplementation with omega–3 fatty acids on plasma fibrinolysis in normal subjects. Thromb Res 1985;39:307–312.
63   Radack K, Deck C, Huster G: Dietary supplementation with low-dose fish oils lowers fibrinogen levels: A randomized, double-blind controlled study. Ann Intern Med 1989;111:757–758.
64   Sanders TAB, Vickers M, Haines AP: Effect on blood lipids and hemostasis of a supplement of cod-liver oil, rich in eicosapentaenoic and docosahexaenoic acids, in healthy young men. Clin Sci 1981;61:317–324.

65   Brown AJ, Roberts DCK: Fish and fish oil intake: effect on hematological variables related to cardiovascular disease. Thromb Res 1991;64:169–178.

66   De Caterina R, Giannessi D, Mazzone A, et al: Vascular prostacyclin is increased in patients ingesting n-3 polyunsaturated fatty acids prior to coronary artery bypass surgery. Circulation 1990;82:428–438.

67   Fox PL, Dicorleto PE: Fish oils inhibit endothelial cell production of a platelet-derived growth factor-like protein. Science 1988;241:453–456.

68   Shimokawa H, Vanhoutte PM: Dietary cod-liver oil improves endothelium dependent responses in hypercholesterolemic and atherosclerotic porcine coronary arteries. Circulation 1988;78: 1421–1430.

69   Kremer JM Jubiz W, Michalek A: Fish-oil fatty acid supplementation in active rheumatoid arthritis. Ann Intern Med 1987;106:497–503.

70   Lee TH, Hoover RL, Williams JD, et al: Effect of dietary enrichment with eicosapentaenoic and docosahexaenoic acids on in vitro neutrophil and monocyte leukotriene generation and neutrophil function. N Engl J Med 1985;312:1217–1224.

71   Endres S, Ghorbani R, Kelley VE, et al: The effect of dietary supplementation with n-3 polyunsaturated fatty acids on the synthesis of interleukin-1 and tumor necrosis factor by mononuclear cells. N Engl J Med 1989;320:265–271.

72   Khalfoun B, Thibault F, Watier H, Bardos P, Lebranchu Y: Docosahexaenoic and eicosapentaenoic acids inhibit in vitro human endothelial cell production of interleukin-6; in Honn KV, et al (eds): Eicosanoids and Other Bioactive Lipids in Cancer, Inflammation, and Radiation Injury 2. New York, Plenum Press, 1997.

73   Kremer JM, Lawrence DA, Jubiz W: Different doses of fish-oil fatty acid ingestion in active rheumatoid arthritis: A prospective study of clinical and immunological parameters; in Galli C, Simopoulos AP (eds): Dietary ω3 and ω6 Fatty Acids: Biological Effects and Nutritional Essentiality. New York, Plenum Publishing, 1989, pp 343–350.

74   Robinson DR, Kremer JM: Summary of Panel G: rheumatoid arthritis and inflammatory mediators; in Simopoulos AP, Kifer RR, Martin RE, Barlow SM (eds): Health Effects of ω3 Polyunsaturated Fatty Acids in Seafoods. World Rev Nutr Diet. Basel, Karger, 1991, vol 66, pp 44–47.

75   Ross R: Atherosclerosis: An inflammatory disease. N Engl J Med 1999;340:115–126.

76   Springer TA: Traffic signals for lymphocyte recirculation and leukocyte emigration: The multistep paradigm. Cell 1994;76:301–314.

77   Davies MJ, Gordon JL, Gearing AJH, Pigott R, Woolf N, Katz D, Kyriakopoulos A: The expression of the adhesion molecules ICAM-1, VCAM-1, PECAM, and E-selectin in human atherosclerosis. J Pathol 1993;171:223–229.

78   O'Brien KD, Allen MD, McDonald TO, Chait A, Harlan JM, Fishbein D, McCarty J, Ferguson M, Hudkins K, Benjamin CD: Vascular cell adhesion molecule-1 is expressed in human coronary atherosclerotic plaques: implications for the mode of progression of advanced coronary atherosclerosis. J Clin Invest 1993;92:945–951.

79   Poston RN, Haskard DO, Coucher JR, Gall NP, Johnson-Tidey RR: Expression of intercellular adhesion molecule-1 in atherosclerotic plaques. Am J Pathol 1992;140:665–673.

80   Richardson M, Hadcock SJ, DeReske M, Cybulsky MI: Increased expression in vivo of VCAM-1 and E-selectin by the aortic endothelium of normolipemic and hyperlipemic diabetic rabbits. Arterioscler Thromb 1994;14:760–769.

81   Simopoulos AP: The role of fatty acids in gene expression: Health implications. Ann Nutr Metab 1996;40:303–311.

82   Ge Y-L, Chen Z, Kang ZB, Cluette-Brown J, Laposata M, Kang JX: Effects of adenoviral transfer of Caenorhabditis elegans n-3 fatty acid desaturase on the lipid profile and growth of human breast cancer cells. Anticancer Res 2002;22:537–544.

83   Kang ZB, Ge Y, Chen Z, Brown J, Lapasota M, Leaf A, Kang JX: Adenoviral transfer of Caenorhabditis elegans n-3 fatty acid desaturase optimizes fatty acid composition in mammalian heart cells. Proc Natl Acad Sci USA 2001;98:4050–4054.

84   De Lorgeril M, Salen P: Dietary prevention of coronary heart disease: Focus on omega–6/ omega–3 essential fatty acid balance. World Rev Nutr Diet. Basel, Karger, 2003, vol 92, pp 57–73.

85 Zampelas A, Paschos G, Rallidis L, Yiannakouris N: Linoleic acid to Alpha-linolenic acid ratio: From clinical trials to inflammatory markers of coronary artery disease. World Rev Nutr Diet. Basel, Karger, 2003, vol 92, pp 92–108.

86 Yehuda S: Omega–6/omega–3 ratio and brain-related functions. World Rev Nutr Diet. Basel, Karger, 2003, vol 92, pp 37–56.

87 Chajes V, Bougnoux P: Omega–6/omega–3 polyunsaturated fatty acid ratio and cancer. World Rev Nutr Diet. Basel, Karger, 2003, vol 92, pp 133–151.

88 Cleland LS, James MJ, Proudman SM: Omega–6/omega–3 fatty acids and arthritis. World Rev Nutr Diet. Basel, Karger, 2003, vol 92, pp 152–168.

89 Maes M, Smith R, Christophe A, Cosyns P, Desnyder R, Meltzer H: Fatty acid composition in major depression: decreased omega 3 fractions in cholesteryl esters and increased C20:4 omega 6/C20:5 omega 3 ratio in cholesteryl esters and phospholipids. J Affect Disord 1996;38:35–46.

90 Maes M, Smith R, Christophe A, Vandoolaeghe E, Van Gastel A, Neels H, Demedts P, Wauters A, Meltzer HY: Lower serum high-density lipoprotein cholesterol (HDL-C) in major depression and in depressed men with serious suicidal attempts: relationship with immune-inflammatory markers. Acta Psychiatr Scand 1997;95:212–221.

91 Peet M, Murphy B, Shay J, Horrobin D: Depletion of omega–3 fatty acid levels in red blood cell membranes of depressive patients. Biol Psychiatry 1998;43:315–319.

92 Locke CA, Stoll AL: Omega–3 fatty acids in major depression. World Rev Nutr Diet. Basel, Karger, 2001, vol 89, pp 173–185.

93 Stoll AL, Severus WE, Freeman MP, Rueter S, Zboyan HA, Diamond E, Cress KK, Marangell LB: Omega 3 fatty acids in bipolar disorder: A preliminary double-blind, placebo-controlled trial. Arch Gen Psychiatry 1999;56:407–412.

94 Simopoulos AP: N-3 fatty acids and human health: Defining strategies for public policy. Lipids 2001;36:S83–S89.

Artemis P. Simopoulos, MD
The Center for Genetics, Nutrition and Health
2001 S Street, N.W., Suite 530, Washington, DC 20009 (USA)
Tel. +1 202 462 5062, Fax +1 202 462 5241, E-Mail cgnh@bellatlantic.net

Appendix I

Recommended Dietary Intakes for Omega–6 and Omega–3 Fatty Acids

On April 7–9, 1999, an international working group of scientists met at the National Institutes of Health in Bethesda, Md., USA to discuss the scientific evidence relative to dietary recommendations of omega–6 and omega–3 fatty acids [Simopoulos, et al., 1999]. The latest scientific evidence based on controlled intervention trials in infant nutrition, cardiovascular disease, and mental health was extensively discussed. Tables 1 and 2 include the Adequate Intakes (AI) for omega–6 and omega–3 essential fatty acids for adults and infant formula/diet, respectively.

Adults

The working group recognized that there are not enough data to determine Dietary Reference Intakes (DRI), but there are good data to make recommendations for Adequate Intakes (AI) for adults as shown in table 1.

Table 1. Adequate intakes (AI)* for adults

Fatty acid	Grams/day (2,000 kcal diet)	% energy
LA	4.44	2.0
(upper limit)[1]	6.67	3.0
ALA	2.22	1.0
DHA + EPA	0.65	0.3
DHA to be at least[2]	0.22	0.1
EPA to be at least	0.22	0.1
TRANS-FA		
(upper limit)[3]	2.00	1.0
SAT		
(upper limit)[4]	–	<8.0
MONOs[5]	–	–

[1]Although the recommendation is for AI, the Working Group felt that there is enough scientific evidence to also state an upper limit (UL) for LA of 6.67 g/day based on a 2,000-kcal diet or of 3.0% of energy.

[2]For pregnant and lactating women, ensure 300 mg/day of DHA.

[3]Except for dairy products, other foods under natural conditions do not contain trans-FA. Therefore, the Working Group does not recommend trans-FA to be in the food supply as a result of hydrogenation of unsaturated fatty acids or high temperature cooking (reused frying oils).

[4]Saturated fats should not comprise more than 8% of energy.

[5]The Working Group recommended that the majority of fatty acids are obtained from monounsaturates. The total amount of fat in the diet is determined by the culture and dietary habits of people around the world (total fat ranges from 15 to 40% of energy) but with special attention to the importance of weight control and reduction of obesity.

*If sufficient scientific evidence is not available to calculate an Estimated Average Requirement, a reference intake called an Adequate Intake is used instead of a Recommended Dietary Allowance. The AI is a value based on experimentally derived intake levels or approximations of observed mean nutrient intakes by a group (or groups) of healthy people. The AI for children and adults is expected to meet or exceed the amount needed to maintain a defined nutritional state or criterion of adequacy in essentially all members of a specific healthy population; LA = Linoleic acid; ALA = alpha-linolenic acid; DHA = docosahexaenoic acid; EPA = eicosapentaenoic acid; TRANS-FA = *trans* fatty acids; SAT = saturated fatty acids; MONOs = monounsaturated fatty acids.

Table 2. AI* for infant formula/diet

Fatty acid	Percent of fatty acids
LA[1]	10.00
ALA	1.50
AA[2]	0.50
DHA	0.35
EPA[3]	
(upper limit)	<0.10

[1]The Working Group recognizes that in countries like Japan, the breast milk content of LA is 6–10% of fatty acids and the DHA is higher, about 0.6%. The formula/diet composition described here is patterned on infant formula studies in Western countries.

[2]The Working Group endorsed the addition of the principal long chain polyunsaturates, AA and DHA, to all infant formulas.

[3]EPA is a natural constituent of breast milk, but in amounts more than 0.1% in infant formula may antagonize AA and interfere with infant growth.

*If sufficient scientific evidence is not available to calculate an Estimated Average Requirement, a reference intake called an Adequate Intake is used instead of a Recommended Dietary Allowance. The AI is a value based on experimentally derived intake levels or approximations of observed mean nutrient intakes by a group (or groups) of healthy people. The AI for children and adults is expected to meet or exceed the amount needed to maintain a defined nutritional state or criterion of adequacy in essentially all members of a specific healthy population. LA = Linoleic acid; ALA = alpha-linolenic acid; AA = arachidonic acid; DHA = docosahexaenoic acid; EPA = eicosapentaenoic acid; TRANS-FA = *trans* fatty acids; SAT = saturated fatty acids; MONOs = monounsaturated fatty acids.

Pregnancy and Lactation

For pregnancy and lactation, the recommendations are the same as those for adults with the additional recommendation seen in footnote 1 (table 2), that during pregnancy and lactation women must ensure a DHA intake of 300 mg/day.

Composition of Infant Formula/Diet

It was thought of utmost importance to focus on the composition of the infant formula considering the large number of premature infants around the world, the low number of women who breast-feed, and the need for proper nutrition of the sick infant. The composition of the infant formula/diet was based on studies that demonstrated support for both the growth and neural development of infants in a manner similar to that of the breast-fed infant (table 2).

One recommendation deserves explanation here. After much discussion consensus was reached on the importance of reducing the omega–6 polyunsaturated fatty acids (PUFAs) even as the omega–3 PUFAs are increased in the diet of adults and newborns for optimal brain and cardiovascular health and function. This is necessary to reduce adverse effects of excesses of arachidonic acid and its eicosanoid products. Such excesses can occur when too much LA and AA are present in the diet and an adequate supply of dietary omega–3 fatty acids is not available. The adverse effects of too much arachidonic acid and its eicosanoids can be avoided by two interdependent dietary changes. First, the amount of plant oils rich in LA, the parent compound of the omega–6 class, which is converted to AA, needs to be reduced. Second, simultaneously the omega–3 PUFAs need to be increased in the diet. LA can be converted to arachidonic acid and the enzyme, delta–6 desaturase, necessary to desaturate it, is the same one necessary to desaturate ALA, the parent compound of the omega–3 class; each competes with the other for this desaturase. The presence of ALA in the diet can inhibit the conversion of the large amounts of LA in the diets of Western industrialized countries which contain too much dietary plant oils rich in omega–6 PUFAs (e.g. corn, safflower, and soybean oils). The increase of ALA, together with EPA and DHA, and reduction of vegetable oils with high LA content, are necessary to achieve a healthier diet in these countries.

Simopoulos AP, Cleland LG (eds): Omega–6/Omega–3 Essential Fatty Acid Ratio:
The Scientific Evidence. World Rev Nutr Diet. Basel, Karger, 2003, vol 92, pp 23–36

....

The Importance of Omega–6/ Omega–3 Fatty Acid Ratio in Cell Function

The Gene Transfer of Omega–3 Fatty Acid Desaturase

Jing X. Kang

Massachusetts General Hospital and Harvard Medical School,
Boston, Mass., USA

Recent research has shown that omega–3 polyunsaturated fatty acids (omega–3 PUFA) have many health-promoting, disease-preventing or medicinal properties [1–3]. From epidemiology to cell culture and animal studies to randomized controlled trials, numerous beneficial effects, including the cardio-protective effect [4–6], anti-inflammatory effect [7–9] and anticancer effect [10–12], of omega–3 fatty acids are becoming recognized. It has been suggested that the therapeutic or preventive efficacy of omega–3 PUFA depends not only on the absolute amount of omega–3 PUFA available but also on the proportion of omega–3 PUFA to the background levels of omega–6 PUFA in cells [13–15], because these two classes of PUFA (omega–6 and omega–3) are metabolically and functionally distinct (antagonistic). In general, excessive amounts of omega–6 PUFA and a very high omega–6/omega–3 ratio promote the patho-genesis of many diseases, including inflammatory disorders, cancer and cardio-vascular disease, whereas increased levels of omega–3 PUFA (a low omega–6/omega–3 ratio) exert suppressive effects [1–3, 13–15]. Thus, it seems that the ratio of omega–6 to omega–3 fatty acids, other than absolute quantity of omega–3 fatty acids, plays a critical role in the prevention and treatment of many clinical problems.

According to recent studies [16], the ratio of omega–6 to omega–3 essen-tial fatty acids in today's Western diets is around 15–20:1, indicating that modern diets are deficient in omega–3 fatty acids but too high in omega–6 fatty

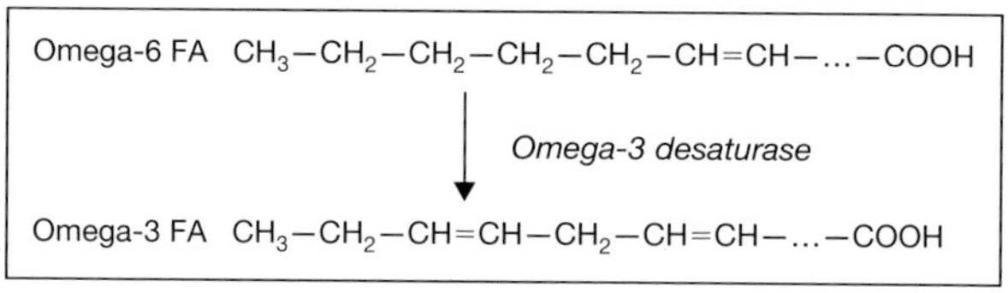

Fig. 1. Conversion of omega–6 fatty acids (FA) to omega–3 fatty acids by an omega–3 desaturase that does not exist in mammalian cells. The omega–3 desaturase can catalyze introduction of a double bond into omega–6 fatty acids at the omega–3 position of their hydrocarbon chains to form omega–3 fatty acids.

acids compared with the diet on which humans evolved and their genetic patterns were established (omega–6/omega–3 was 1:1) [17]. The lipid pattern of our diets renders our tissues very high in omega–6 PUFA (a high omega–6/omega–3 ratio). The high omega–6/omega–3 ratio may contribute to the high prevalence of many modern diseases (e.g. heart disease, cancer). It is hypothesized that balancing or reducing the ratio of omega–6/omega–3 fatty acids may decrease the risk of these diseases. At the molecular level, converting the excessive omega–6 PUFA to omega–3 PUFA may have beneficial effects on cell function. However, mammalian cells naturally cannot convert omega–6 PUFA to omega–3 PUFA because they lack the gene encoding a converting enzyme, namely, omega–3 fatty acid desaturase. Nevertheless, such an enzyme exists in *Caenorhabditis elegans* (round worm). The gene, namely *fat-1*, encoding the omega–3 desaturase has recently been cloned from the organism [18]. Functionally, the omega–3 desaturase can introduce a double bond into omega–6 fatty acids at the omega–3 position of their hydrocarbon chains to form omega–3 fatty acids (see fig. 1, for illustration). Therefore, it is possible to modify cellular omega–6/omega–3 fatty acid ratio by expression of the *C. elegans* omega–3 desaturase in mammalian cells. We have recently explored this possibility in several cell types and proven this genetic approach uniquely effective in balancing the cellular omega–6/omega–3 fatty acid ratio [19–22]. In comparison with supplementation, the gene transfer approach is superior in balancing the omega–6/omega–3 fatty acid ratio because it not only enhances absolute quantity of omega–3 PUFA but also simultaneously decreases the level of omega–6 PUFA. Unlike the supplementation with exogenous fatty acids, this gene transfer approach needs no incorporation of exogenous fatty acids into cells to alter the omega–6/omega–3 ratio and therefore does not change the total amount of cellular fatty acids (i.e. no difference in lipid mass between treated cells and control cells). Thus, the transgenic cells created by this technology can serve as a unique model for elucidating the significance of the ratio of omega–6 to omega–3 PUFA.

Kang

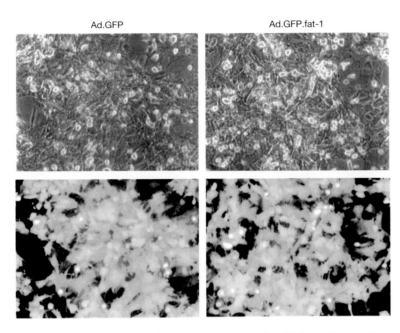

Ad.GFP   Ad.GFP.fat-1

Fig. 2. Photomicrographs showing gene transfer efficiency. Rat cardiac myocytes were infected with Ad.GFP (left panels; control) or Ad.GFP.fat-1 (right panels). Forty-eight hours after infection, cardiomyocytes were visualized with bright light (upper panels) and at 510 nm of blue light (lower panels). Co-expression of GFP demonstrates visually that the transgene is being expressed in cells in a high efficiency.

Heterologous Expression of *C. elegans* Omega–3 Fatty Acid Desaturase in Mammalian Cells

In order to introduce the *fat-1* gene into mammalian cells efficiently, we used a virus-mediated gene transfer strategy. We constructed a recombinant adenovirus (Ad.GFP.fat-1) carrying both the *fat-1* gene and the GFP gene (green fluorescent protein gene) and another adenovirus (Ad.GFP) carrying the GFP gene alone (as control) and used them to infect various mammalian cells, including heart cells, neurons, endothelial cells and human breast cancer cells [19–22]. The co-expression of GFP allows us to identify cells that are infected and express the transgene. Figure 2 shows the efficiency of the adenovirus-mediated gene transfer in cultured cardiac myocytes. Forty-eight hours after infection, the majority (>90%) of cells exhibited bright fluorescence, indicating a high efficiency of gene transfer and a high expression level of the transgene. The expression profile of the transgene (*fat-1*) was also determined by mRNA analysis using ribonuclease protection assay. As shown in figure 3,

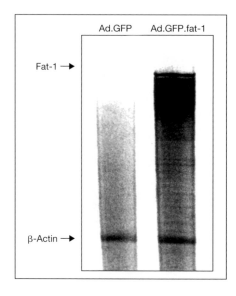

Fig. 3. Ribonuclease protection assay of fat-1 transcript levels in cells infected with Ad.GFP (control) and myocytes infected with Ad.GFP.fat-1. Total RNA (10 μg) isolated from the cells was hybridized with anti-sense RNA probes, digested with RNase and resolved in denaturing PAGE gel. The fat-1mRNA was visualized by autoradiography. A probe targeting-actin gene was used as control.

fat-1 mRNA was highly abundant in cells infected with the adenovirus carrying the *fat-1* gene, but was not detected at all in cells infected with the control adenovirus [19–22]. This result indicates that the adenovirus-mediated gene transfer could confer very high expression of *fat-1* gene in mammalian cells, which normally lack the gene.

Biochemical Effects

To determine if the expression of the *fat-1* gene in mammalian cells could change their lipid profile, cellular lipids were extracted and fatty acid composition was analyzed by gas chromatography-mass spectrometry. Our results showed that the fatty acid profiles were remarkably different between cells expressing the *fat-1* gene and control cells [19–22]. Figure 4 shows the differences of cellular fatty acid profiles in cardiac myocytes. In cells expressing the *fat-1* gene (omega–3 fatty acid desaturase), all types of omega–6 fatty acids were largely converted to corresponding omega–3 fatty acids, namely 18:2ω6 to 18:3ω3, 20:2ω6 to 20:3ω3, 20:3ω6 to 20:4ω3, 20:4ω6 to 20:5ω3, 22:4ω6 to 22:5ω3 and 22:5ω6 to 22:6ω3 (fig. 4). As a result, the fatty acid composition of the cells expressing *fat-1* gene was significantly changed when compared to that of the control cells. Importantly, the ratio of omega–6/omega–3 was dramatically reduced from 9–15:1 in the control

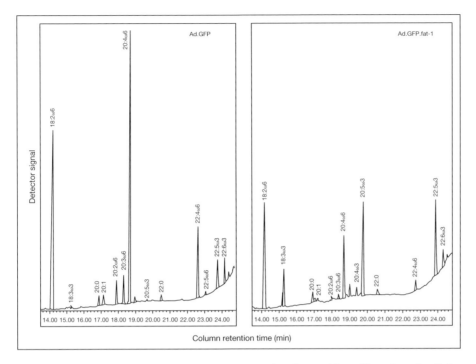

Fig. 4. Partial gas chromatograph traces showing fatty acid profiles of total cellular lipids extracted from cultured neonatal rat cardiac myocytes infected with Ad.GFP (control) and the myocytes infected with Ad.GFP.fat-1.

cells to about 1:1 in the cells expressing the omega–3 fatty acid desaturase (table 1). Similar effects were observed in other cell types that we have tested [20–22]. Obviously, the *fat-1* gene can be functionally expressed in mammalian cells, and its expression can exerts a remarkable effect on cellular fatty acid composition.

To examine whether the gene transfer-induced alteration in the ratio of omega–6 to omega–3 can lead to a change in the profile of eicosanoids generated by the cells, we measured the production of prostaglandin E_2 (PGE$_2$), one of the major ecosanoids derived from 20:4ω6 (AA), by using an enzyme immunoassay [19–21]. As expected, the amount of prostaglandin E_2 produced by the cells expressing the *fat-1* gene was significantly lower than that produced by the control cells (30–50% reduction) [19–21]. A representative set of data indicating the change in cardiac myocytes is shown in figure 5. Our data indicate that the gene transfer can effectively modulate the generation of eicosanoids.

Table 1. Polyunsaturated fatty acid composition of total cellular lipids from the control heart cells and the transgenic cells expressing a *C. elegans fat-1* cDNA

mol% of total fatty acids	Control	*fat-1*
ω6 Polyunsaturates		
18:2ω6	14.2[a]	9.2[b]
20:2ω6	1.2[a]	0.3[b]
20:3ω6	1.6[a]	0.4[b]
20:4ω6	15.2[a]	4.1[b]
22:4ω6	4.4[a]	1.0[b]
22:5ω6	0.2[a]	0.0[b]
Total	36.8[a]	15.0[b]
ω3 Polyunsaturates		
18:3ω3	0.2[b]	3.6[a]
20:4ω3	0.0[b]	0.6[a]
20:5ω3	0.1[b]	6.1[a]
22:5ω3	1.2[b]	5.8[a]
22:6ω3	1.0[a]	1.3[a]
Total	2.5[b]	17.4[a]
ω6/ω3 ratio	14.7[a]	0.9[b]

Values are means of four measurements. Values for each fatty acid with the same letter do not differ significantly ($p < 0.01$) between control and fat-1.

Physiological Effects

To determine if the gene transfer-induced change in the omega–6/omega–3 ratio would provide the beneficial effects of omega–3 fatty acids as observed with fatty acid supplementation, we have examined physiological responses in different cell types after gene transfer.

Our previous studies have demonstrated an antiarrhythmic effect for omega–3 fatty acids when supplemented to cardiac myocytes [23]. To see whether the gene transfer can provide a similar protective effect, neonatal rat cardiac myocytes expressing the *fat-1* gene were tested for their susceptibility to arrhythmias induced by arrhythmogenic agents, such as high concentrations of extracellular calcium. As shown in figure 6, when challenged with a high $[Ca^{2+}]$ (7.5 mM), the control cells promptly exhibited arrhythmia characterized by spasmodic contractures and fibrillation, whereas the cells expressing the *fat-1* gene could sustain regular beating (resistant to the arrhythmogenic stimulus),

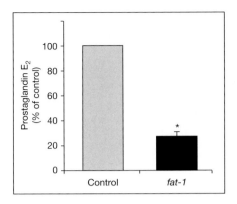

Fig. 5. Enzyme immunoassay of prostaglandin E_2 levels in the control cells and the cells expressing the *fat-1* gene. Values are means SD of three experiments and expressed as % of control. *$p < 0.01$.

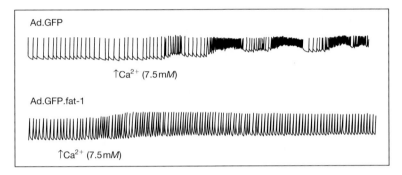

Fig. 6. Effect of expression of the *C. elegans* omega–3 fatty acid desaturase in cardiac myocytes on their susceptibility to arrhythmia. Cultured (spontaneously beating) neonatal rat cardiac myocytes infected with Ad.GFP (control) or Ad.GFP.fat-1 were challenged with 7.5 mM extracellular calcium. The control cells promptly exhibited arrhythmia (spasmodic contractures and fibrillation), whereas the *fat-1* cells could sustain regular beating.

similar to the effect of omega–3 fatty acid supplementation [23]. This suggests that gene transfer of the omega–3 desaturase into heart cells can provide the antiarrhythmic effect of omega–3 fatty acids.

In human breast cancer cells (MCF-7), gene transfer of the omega–3 desaturase reduced both cellular omega–6/omega–3 fatty acid ratio from 12.0 to 0.8 and the level of PGE_2 by about 40%, leading to an increase in apoptotic cell death and a decrease in cell proliferation [20]. As shown in figure 7, a large number of the cells expressing *fat-1* gene underwent apoptosis, as indicated by morphological changes (small size with round shape or fragmentation) and nuclear staining (bright blue). Statistical analysis of apoptotic cell counts

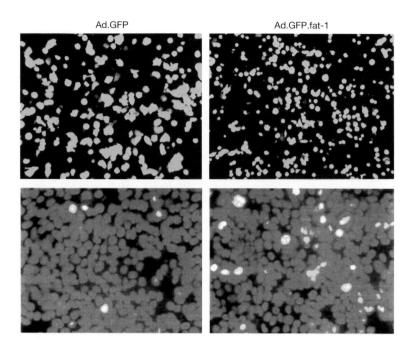

Ad.GFP   Ad.GFP.fat-1

Fig. 7. The gene transfer induces apoptosis of MCF-7 cells. MCF-7 cells were infected with Ad.GFP (left; control) or Ad.GFP.fat-1 (right). Three days after infection, cell death was examined using a fluorescence microscope. Upper panels: Infected cells were directly visualized at 510 nm of blue light. Lower panels: Cells were stained with Hoechst dye for nuclei and observed under 480 nm fluorescent light. The brighter blue spots are the nuclei of apoptotic cells.

showed that 30–50% of cells infected with Ad.GFP.fat-1 were apoptotic whereas only 10% dead cells found in the control cells (infected with Ad.GFP) (fig. 8a). MTT analysis indicated that proliferative activity of cells infected with Ad.GFP.fat-1 was significantly lower than that of cells infected with Ad.GFP (fig. 8b). Accordingly, the total number of viable cells in the cells infected with Ad.GFP.fat-1 was about 30% less than that in the control cells. In an in vivo experiment, nude mice bearing human breast cancer xenografts (MDA-MB-231) were injected intratumorally with the recombinant adenovirus carrying the *fat-1* gene. Over a treatment period of 4 weeks, the growth rate of the tumors treated with the *fat-1* gene was much slower when compared with that of the control tumors injected with the control vector [unpubl. data]. Interestingly, our preliminary data derived from DNA microarray assays showed that the gene transfer-induced change in omega–6/omega–3 fatty acid ratio could result in a downregulation of a number of genes involved in cell proliferation, adhesion, angiogenesis and invasion, with an upregulation of

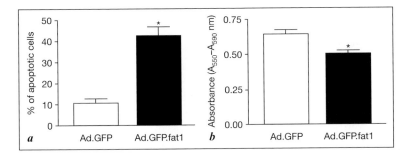

Fig. 8. Effect of the gene transfer on the growth and death of MCF-7 cells. After infection of MCF-7 cells with Ad.GFP (control) or Ad.GFP.fat-1 for 3 days, the percentage of apoptotic cells (*a*) was determined by nuclear staining (as described in fig. 4). The cell proliferation (*b*) was assessed by MTT assay. n = 4, *p < 0.01.

apoptosis-inducing genes in MDA-MB-231 cells [unpubl. data]. These results are consistent with the reported anti-cancer effects of omega–3 fatty acid supplementation [10–12].

In primary culture of human umbilical vein endothelial cells (HUVEC), expression of *fat-1* significantly reduced omega–6/omega–3 fatty acid ratio from about 9 to 1 [22]. This change in cellular omega–6/omega–3 ratio led to a decrease in the surface expression of adhesion molecules (markers of inflammation). As shown in figure 9, the quantity of the adhesion molecules (as determined by immunoassay), E-selectin, ICAM-1, and VCAM-1 was reduced by 42, 43 and 57%, respectively, in response to cytokine exposure (TNF-α 5 U/ml, 4 h) [22]. We (in collaboration with Dr. Anthony Rosenzweig) then examined whether changes in the adhesion molecule profile were sufficient to alter endothelial interactions with monocytes, the most prevalent white blood cell type found in atherosclerotic lesions. Under laminar flow and a defined shear stress of ~2 dyn/cm^2, fat-1 compared to control vector infected HUVEC supported ~50% less firm adhesion with almost no effect on the rolling interactions of THP-1 cells [22]. These results indicate that expression of the *fat-1* gene in HUVEC inhibit cytokine induction of the endothelial inflammatory response and firm adhesion of monocytes, suggesting that a balanced omega–6/omega–3 fatty acid ratio may have an antiatherosclerotic effect.

We have also determined the effect of *fat-1* expression on neuronal apoptosis. We found that the expression of the *fat-1* gene, which could significantly reduce the neuronal omega–6/omega–3 fatty acid ratio from 6 to 1.5 and the production of prostaglandin E$_2$ by 20%, resulted in protection from growth factor-withdrawal-induced apoptotic cell death of rat cortical neurons [21]. Following gene transfer, apoptosis was induced by 24 h of growth factor

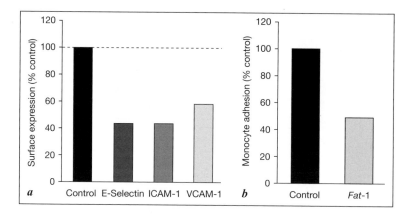

Fig. 9. Effect of the gene transfer on the surface expression of adhesion molecules (*a*) and the interaction with monocytes (*b*) in human umbilical vein endothelial cells (HUVEC). Monolayers of primary HUVEC were infected with Ad.GFP.fat-1 or the control Ad.GFP for 36 h, exposed for 4 h to the cytokine TNF-α, and subjected to immunoassay analysis for surface adhesion molecules and videomicroscopy to examine endothelial interactions with the monocytic cell line, THP-1, under laminar flow conditions. The bars represent the percentages of control.

withdrawal and detected by Hoechst staining. As shown in figure 10, cortical cultures infected with the Ad.GFP.fat-1 underwent (~60%) less apoptosis than those infected with Ad.GFP [21]. Accordingly, MTT analysis indicated that the viability of Ad.GFP.fat-1 cells was significantly (~50%) higher than that of cells infected with Ad.GFP (fig. 11). The observed protective effect of gene transfer on neuronal apoptosis mimics the protective effects of omega–3 fatty acid supplementation [24, 25] and highlights the importance of omega–6/omega–3 ratio in this neuroprotectve effect.

Implications

Our findings as presented here clearly indicate that virus-mediated gene transfer of the *C. elegans* omega–3 fatty acid desaturase can quickly and dramatically balance the cellular omega–6/omega–3 fatty acid ratio, alter eicosanoid profile, and consequently provide beneficial effects of omega–3 fatty acids, without the need for supplementation with exogenous omega–3 fatty acids. Thus, our studies have demonstrated a novel and effective approach to modifying fatty acid composition of mammalian cells. The high efficacy of this genetic approach in modifying omega–6/omega–3 ratio makes it helpful for studying the importance of omega–6/omega–3 fatty acid ratio in a biological system.

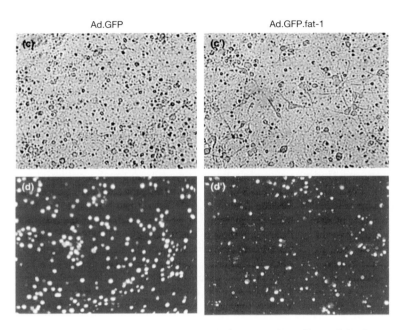

Ad.GFP   Ad.GFP.fat-1

Fig. 10. Photomicrographs showing the protective effect of *fat-1* gene on neuronal apoptosis. Cells were infected with Ad.GFP (left panels, control) or Ad.GFP.fat-1 (right panels). Cell death was examined after 24 h of growth factor withdrawal using a fluorescent microscope. Bright-field (upper panels) and Hoecsht staining (lower panels) images showing apoptotic cells.

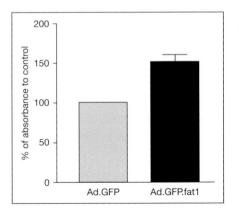

Fig. 11. MTT assay of cell viability in control and *fat-1* expressing cultures. After 24 h of growth factor withdrawal, the cell viability of cells expressing the *fat-1* gene is 50% higher than control cells ($p < 0.01$).

Indeed, our data derived from the omega–3 desaturase gene transfer clearly show that a low or balanced omega–6/omega–3 fatty acid ratio exerts a beneficial effect in different cell types (decreased susceptibility of heart cells to arrhythmia, reduced inflammatory response of endothelial cells, increased apoptosis of cancer cells and enhanced survival of neurons against ischemia). These results strongly support the notion that excessive amounts of omega–6 PUFA and a very high omega–6/omega–3 ratio promote the pathogenesis of many modern diseases (e.g. heart disease, cancer), while balancing or reducing the ratio of omega–6/omega–3 fatty acids may decrease the risk of these diseases. In vivo studies using *fat-1* transgenic mice ('Omega–3' mice, which are being created in our lab) will be more interesting and will give more meaningful and definite information about the importance of a balanced omega–6/omega–3 ratio in disease prevention.

In addition, our findings provide a basis (feasibility) for the potential use of the omega–3 desaturase gene transfer as a gene therapy for patients who are at high risk of life-threatening diseases such as cardiovascular disease and cancer. Potentially, this approach will become an alternative therapy for patients with advanced disease or those who fail to pursue ingestion of supplements or a change in dietary habits.

Furthermore, our findings provide a new strategy for producing omega–3 PUFA-enriched foodstuff (e.g. meat, milk and eggs) by generating large transgenic animals (e.g. cow, pig, sheep and chicken) with the omega–3 desaturase gene. In recognition of the health benefits of omega–3 fatty acids and the deficiency of these fatty acids in Western diets, a great effort has now been made to return omega–3 fatty acids into the food supply [26]. Since most animals can not produce omega–3 fatty acids themselves, what the food industry is currently doing in order to enrich animal food products with omega–3 fatty acids is to feed animals with flax seed, fish meal or other marine products. This feeding procedure is not only time consuming and costly, but source-limited. Thus, the feeding strategy seems to be an unsustainable way of producing omega–3 enriched foodstuff. With the use of our gene transfer strategy, transgenic animals (e.g. cow, pig, sheep and chicken) genetically capable of producing omega–3 fatty acids themselves can be created. This, therefore, can eliminate the need of lengthy feeding with omega–3 fatty acid-containing diets. Obviously, the 'Omega–3' transgenic animals may probably serve as a new and promising resource to meet the increasing demand for omega–3 essential fatty acids.

Acknowledgements

We thank Dr. John Browse for generously providing the *C. elegans fat-1* cDNA. We are grateful to Dr. Alexander Leaf for his general support and helpful discussions. This work was supported by National Institute Grant CA79553, the Harvard Clinical Research Center/NIH Grant #P30 DK40561 and the American Institute for Cancer Research Grant 2A-017 (to *J.X.K.*).

References

1   Connor WE: Importance of n–3 fatty acids in health and disease. Am J Clin Nutr 2000;71: 171S–175S.
2   Simopoulos AP: Essential fatty acids in health and chronic disease. Am J Clin Nutr 1999; 70:560S–569S.
3   Salem N Jr, Simopoulos AP, Galli C, Lagarde M, Knapp HR: Fatty acids and lipids from cell biology to human disease. Lipids 1996;31(suppl):S1–S326.
4   Leaf A, Kang JX: Omega 3 fatty acids and cardiovascular disease. World Rev Nutr Diet. Basel, Karger, 1998, vol 83, pp 24–37.
5   De Caterina R, Endres S, Kristensen SD, Schmidt EB: n–3 Fatty Acids and Vascular Disease. London, Springer, 1999, pp 1–166.
6   O'Keefe JH Jr, Harris WS: From inuit to implementation: Omega–3 fatty acids come of age. Mayo Clin Proc 2000;75:607–614.
7   Kelley DS: Modulation of human immune and inflammatory responses by dietary fatty acids. Nutrition 2001;17:669–673.
8   Kremer JM: n–3 fatty acid supplements in rheumatoid arthritis. Am J Clin Nutr 2000;71: 349S–351S.
9   James MJ, Gibson RA, Cleland LG: Dietary polyunsaturated fatty acids and inflammatory mediator production. Am J Clin Nutr 2000;71:343S–348S.
10 Bougnoux P: N–3 polyunsaturated fatty acids and cancer. Curr Opin Clin Nutr Metab Care 1999; 2:121–126.
11 Cave WT Jr: Omega–3 polyunsaturated fatty acids in rodent models of breast cancer. Breast Cancer Res Treat 1997;46:239–246.
12 Rose DP, Connolly JM: Omega–3 fatty acids as cancer chemopreventive agents. Pharmacol Ther 1999;83:217–244.
13 Simonsen N, van't Veer P, Strain JJ, Martin-Moreno JM, Huttunen JK, Navajas JF, Martin BC, Thamm M, Kardinaal AFM, Kok FJ, Kohlmeier L: Adipose tissue omega–3 and omega–6 fatty acid content and breast cancer in the EURAMIC study. Am J Epidemiol 1998;147:342–352.
14 Okuyama H, Kobayashi T, Watanabe S: Dietary fatty acids – the n–6/n–3 balance and chronic elderly diseases: Excess linoleic acid and relative n–3 deficiency syndrome seen in Japan. Prog Lipid Res 1996;35:409–457.
15 Maillard V, Bougnoux P, Ferrari P, Jourdan ML, Pinault M, Lavillonniere F, Body G, Le Floch O, Chajes V: N–3 and N–6 fatty acids in breast adipose tissue and relative risk of breast cancer in a case-control study in Tours, France. Int J Cancer 2002;98:78–83.
16 Simopoulos AP: Human requirement for n–3 polyunsaturated fatty acids. Poultry Sci 2000; 79:961–970.
17 Leaf A, Weber PC: A new era for science in nutrition. Am J Clin Nutr 1987;45:1048–1053.
18 Spychalla JP, Kinney AJ, Browse J: Identification of an animal omega–3 fatty acid desaturase by heterologous expression in arabidopsis. Proc Natl Acad Sci USA 1997;94:1142–1147.
19 Kang ZB, Ge Y, Chen ZH, Brown J, Laposata M, Leaf A, Kang JX: Adenoviral gene transfer of C. elegans n–3 fatty acid desaturase optimizes fatty acid composition in mammalian cells. Proc Natl Acad Sci USA 2001;98:4050–4054.
20 Ge Y, Chen ZH, Brown J, Laposata M, Kang JX: Effect of adenoviral gene transfer of C. elegans n–3 fatty acid desaturase on the lipid profile and growth of human breast cancer cells. Anticancer Res 2002;22:537–544.
21 Ge Y, Wang XY, Chen ZH, Landman N, Lo EH, Kang JX: Inhibition of neuronal apoptosis by adenoviral gene transfer of C. elegans n–3 fatty acid desaturase. J Neurochem 2002;82: 1360–1366.
22 Meiler S, Kang JX, Rosenzweig A: Expression of the fat-1 gene alters lipid profile and inhibits the inflammation of human endothelium by reducing the transcriptional activity of NFkB. American Heart Association Annual Meeting Abstract, 2002, publ ID:1228.
23 Kang JX, Leaf A: Antiarrhythmic effects of polyunsaturated fatty acids: Recent studies. Circulation 1996;94:1774–1780.

24 Kim HY, Akbar M, Lau A, Edsall L: Inhibition of neuronal apoptosis by docosahexaenoic acid (22:6n–3): Role of phosphatidylserine in antiapoptotic effect. J Biol Chem 2000;275: 35215–35223.

25 Lauritzen I, Blondeau N, Heurteaux C, Widmann C, Romey G, Lazdunski M: Polyunsaturated fatty acids are potent neuroprotectors. EMBO J 2000;19:1784–1793.

26 Simopoulos AP, et al (eds): The return of ω3 fatty acids into the food supply: Land-based animal food products and their health effects. World Rev Nutr Diet. Basel, Karger, 1998, vol 83.

Jing X. Kang
Massachusetts General Hospital
149–13th Street, Room 4433, Charlestown, MA 02129 (USA)
Tel. +1 617 726 8509, Fax +1 617 726 6144, E-Mail kang.jing@mgh.harvard.edu

Simopoulos AP, Cleland LG (eds): Omega–6/Omega–3 Essential Fatty Acid Ratio:
The Scientific Evidence. World Rev Nutr Diet. Basel, Karger, 2003, vol 92, pp 37–56

....

Omega–6/Omega–3 Ratio and Brain-Related Functions

Shlomo Yehuda

Psychopharmacology Laboratory, Department of Psychology,
Bar Ilan University, Ramat Gan, Israel

While the general public typically perceives lipids and fats as 'harmful' components of the diet (as in the popular slogan: 'fat kills'), the scientific story is in fact very different.

Among the major scientific research efforts of the recent period, in the area of neuroscience, we find the recognition of the 'essential fatty acids' (EFA). The profound effects of various fatty acids, and equally profound effects of their deficits, are appreciated by a variety of disciplines, including (but not necessarily limited to) lipid biochemistry, physiology, nutrition, psychology, psychiatry, and neurosciences at large. Recently, the issue of lipids, and fatty acids ratio in diets, became an important issue. Simopoulos [1] showed the historical shift from a 'balanced' omega–6 and omega–3 ratio diet, towards a marked and significant reduction in the omega–3 intake, and explained that the general 'Western diet' of today can in actual fact be considered an omega–3-deficient diet. Her concern is that this 'deficiency' may lead to coronary heart disease and high cancer mortality.

Linoleic acid (LA; omega–6; ω6; 18:2ω6) is the parent fatty acid of the omega–6 group. Linoleic acid must be supplied to the body by the diet, because the body is unable to synthesize it. All other members of the omega–6 group are derivatives of LA. Similarly, the parent compound of the omega–3 group is alpha-linolenic acid (ALA, omega–3, ω3, 18:3ω3). All other members of the omega–3 group are merely derivatives of ALA, and together they form the polyunsaturated fatty acids (PUFA). In each group, the derivatives can convert to longer chain fatty acids by using two mechanisms: desaturation and elongation.

The enzymes that are involved in these mechanisms have the same functions in the two fatty acid groups, and therefore the omega–6 and omega–3 fatty acids 'compete' for the same enzymes.

While from a chemical point of view the differences between omega–6 and omega–3 acids are very small, and may appear insignificant, they exert different and sometimes even opposite effects. These opposing effects are not easily explained. It was recently suggested [2] that the distinction between omega–6 and omega–3 PUFA is based on the differential capacity of protein in large, and membrane-bound protein in particular, to 'recognize' various PUFA. The dietary deficiency of omega–3 fatty acids, as well as the particular roles of omega–6 and omega–3, will become obvious as we take a deeper look into the ratio issue.

The Importance of the Ratio

There are several aspects to the issue of the optimal recommended ratio between omega–6 and omega–3 fatty acids. One aspect is the recommendation for total daily dietary intake in various phases of life (e.g. infancy, pregnancy, adulthood and old age). Another aspect is the optimal ratio of PUFA as a food supplement or treatment. PUFA are used in the body in a variety of conditions, such as in dermatological diseases and in cardiovascular disorders. One particular area is the role of PUFA in the brain and the utility of PUFA to protect and stabilize the neuronal membrane in health and in disease. Our comments in this chapter will be limited to PUFA in the central nervous system (CNS) and CNS conditions.

The effects of PUFA on brain function can be divided into at least five categories: (1) modification of neuronal membrane fluidity; (2) modification of membrane activity-bound enzymes; (3) modification of the number and affinity of receptors; (4) modification of the function of neuronal membrane ionic channels, and (5) modification of the production of neurotransmitters and brain peptides [3].

Many studies have demonstrated that various PUFA mediate, or are associated with, several aspects of brain activity, ranging from the role of EFA in neuronal structure and functions, long-term potentiation (LTP), specific brain activation, prostaglandin activity, to neurological and mental disorders, to mood control. Unfortunately, the vast majority of these studies merely test one or two specific fatty acids, and there are very few solid studies that experimentally examine a wide range of ratios between omega–6 and omega–3. The following review will summarize the areas in which studies on ratios were performed, and will subsequently have to leave out some of the most fascinating areas such as depression, psychosis and pain.

Essential Fatty Acids, the Blood-Brain Barrier, and the Brain

Since EFA must be supplied via the diet, two major issues arise:

Firstly, do EFA and PUFA have the possibility to cross the blood-brain barrier (BBB)? Recently, Rapoport [4] and Edmond [5] provided a detailed discussion on the complex mechanism of delivery of essential PUFA, as it progresses from the blood into the brain. In two developmental periods the involvement of the BBB is crucial, i.e. in infancy and in aging. The human infant is born with immature BBB and during these periods the structure and functions of the BBB are not at their optimal levels. There have been reports of structural changes in the BBB complex, in aging and in Alzheimer's patients [6, 7], but despite the knowledge about structural changes, the knowledge of functional changes is quite limited. Most of the studies did not find changes in the rate of transport of PUFA into the brain during aging [e.g. 8, 9]. The important, but so far unanswered question is whether omega–6 and omega–3 fatty acids have different rates of transport into the brain.

The second issue regarding the BBB is the brain's ability to convert linoleic and alpha-linolenic acids into longer chain fatty acids, arachidonic acid (AA) and docosahexaenoic acid (DHA). Some researchers suspect that the immature brain of the infant is unable to convert these fatty acids to longer chain fatty acids. However, the majority of studies agree that even the infant brain indeed does have such capacity [4, 10].

Brain Neurotransmitters and PUFA

The relationships between PUFA ratios and the various neurotransmitters, as described before [11], are of special interest. It is important to note that omega–3 deficiency induced reduction in dopamine vesicle density in the cortex [12], and malfunction of the dopaminegic mesocorticolimbic pathway [13]. The ability to recover from the dopaminergic effects of omega–3 deficiency is age-dependent [14–16]. Also, the effects of alpha-linolenic acid for recovering from omega–3 deficiency is dependent on spatial configuration. The trans-isomer of alpha-linolenic acid is inactive and if not enough *cis*-isomer is supplied, a state of omega–3 deficiency will occur [16]. Some studies indicate similar effects on the serotonergic system [17].

Membrane Fluidity and Myelin

Before considering the effects of PUFA on brain-mediated functions, the effects of PUFA on brain structural components must be elucidated. Fatty acids and lipids are major components in brain structure. Very high levels of fatty acids and lipids can be found in two structural components; in the neuronal membrane and in the myelin sheaths. The neuronal membrane is composed of two lipid layers. The ratio between the proteins and the lipids is about 50–50%, while lipids (about 70%) constitute the majority in the myelin sheaths (about 30%). The protein component is especially stable, while the lipid component has a relatively high turnover rate.

In order to understand the diverse functions, which seem to be mediated by the various PUFA and by the ratio of omega–6 to omega–3, we [18, 19] proposed that the membrane fluidity index is the common denominator for the various effects of PUFA. Some molecules are able to change the physical state (e.g. the fluidity index) of the membrane. For example, alcohol fluidizes the membrane, while cholesterol hardens it. There are two basic questions regarding the hypothesis that PUFA are able to modify the neuronal membrane fluidity index; firstly, whether changes in the lipid component of the neuronal membrane (e.g. different ratio of various fatty acids) would lead to changes in the neuronal functions, and secondly whether supplementation of various fatty acids would affect the composition and the function of the neuronal membrane. A number of studies have shown that EFA supplementation, under certain conditions of composition and time, indeed modifies both the structure and membrane function (summary can be found in Yehuda et al. [20]). (More detailed studies will be described below.)

The integrity of the myelin is of utmost importance for the proper functions of axons in the nervous system. Breakage or lesions in the myelin can lead to disintegration of many of the nervous system functions. Recent studies emphasize the major role of dietary EFA to the normal functions of myelin. Moreover, the EFA are very important in the active phase of the myelin synthesis. If EFA are not available in this phase, or metabolically blocked, amyelination, dysmyelination or demyelination may occur [21, 22]. If EFA deficiency occurs during the postnatal period, a major delay in the myelination process will occur, accompanied by impaired learning, motor, vision, and auditory abnormalities [23]. It is of great interest to note that similar impairments in the myelination process and in the cognitive function can also be found in postnatally iron-deficient rodents and humans [24]. Disorders, which are associated with myelin malfunction or with dysmyelination, can also occur during the adult period. One such disorder is multiple sclerosis. The rate of myelin lipids turnover is age-dependent. The turnover rate is very slow during aging, and therefore the rate of repairing damaged sections of myelin is slower in aging [25].

Prostaglandins

One major issue among the PUFA researchers is what particular fatty acid among the omega–6 or omega–3 PUFA group is preferable to study. On the one hand, some prefer to study linoleic and alpha-linolenic acids, as these are the precursors to all other PUFA molecules and they have a powerful effect on the neuronal membrane. Others prefer to study longer chain fatty acids, as they are the precursors to the special group of prostaglandins.

Essential fatty acids are considered to be a special class of unsaturated fatty acids that also act as precursors of yet other types of fatty acids. Most of the prostaglandins are derivatives of AA (arachidonic acid; itself derived from omega–6) or from DHA (docosahexanoic acid, omega–3) and all of them have a high physiological, hormone-like, activity level. A review on prostaglandins was recently published [19]. The various prostaglandins are involved in numerous brain functions, sometimes with conflicting or opposing effects. Prostaglandins are involved in functions such as regional blood flow and permeability of various biological membranes. It has been suggested that prostaglandins are also involved in the functional level of the activity of cAMP (a second messenger) in the cells. The behavioral and physiological effects of a specific ratio of an omega–6/omega–3 compound (in a ratio of 4:1) correlates with changes in the fatty acid profile and with changes in the cholesterol level [20]. It may well be that such a compound has an effect on the prostaglandin system as well and mediates the behavioral and biochemical changes that have been observed in the rats. There is evidence that prostaglandin D_2 has a profound beneficial effect on sleep. On the other hand, other prostaglandins enhance CRF (corticotropin-releasing factor) activity, which enhances wakefulness. CRF, in turn, induces the release of prostaglandins. Prostaglandins also enhance TRH (thyrotropin-releasing hormone) release, and stimulate the dopaminergic and noradrenergic receptor activity, while beta-endorphin inhibits the prostaglandin synthesis [11]. Very few studies examine the effect of different ratios on production and/or activity of various prostaglandins.

Cholesterol and Fatty Acids

The membrane fluidity index is dependent on two major factors: (1) the level and the composition and percentage of PUFA in the membrane, and

(2) the level of membrane cholesterol. An increase in the PUFA level will result in fluidizing of the neuronal membrane, while an increase in cholesterol will harden the membrane. The membrane should be at an optimal physiological gel state. Therefore, cholesterol, which is a complex lipid, is involved in many functions in the membrane. It is well established that cholesterol decreases the membrane fluidity index, which affects the activity of ion channels and receptor functions, as well as the dopamine release. Moreover, cholesterol is a key molecule in the end product of the CRF-ACTH (adreno-cortico-tropic-hormone) axis. Considering that steroids are derivatives of cholesterol, it is of great interest to find that various fatty acids have differential effects on cholesterol metabolism. Many reliable studies confirm that the administration of omega–6 fatty acids reduces the level of cholesterol in the blood. However, omega–6 fatty acids and omega–3 fatty acids differ in their mode of action in cholesterol reduction, such that omega–6 fatty acids redistribute cholesterol while the omega–3 fatty acids actually reduce the level of cholesterol in the neuronal membrane. This may explain why an increase in the cholesterol level in the blood is found in humans who consume omega–3 fatty acid supplements. It has been demonstrated that omega–3 essential fatty acids are more effective in reducing cholesterol levels in macrophages than omega–6 essential fatty acids. This is most probably due to the differential effect on the enzyme acyl-coenzyme A activity. However, some studies have indicated that cholesterol-esterifying enzymes that incorporate free fatty acids into cholesterol esters, without the participation of CoA, are also present in the rat brain [26].

The mechanism by which omega–6 or omega–3 fatty acids are able to reduce the cholesterol level in the blood or in the neuronal membrane is still unclear, although several hypotheses have been proposed. For example, Bourre et al. [27] claimed that alpha-linolenic acid controls the composition of nerve membranes, which implies an inverse relationship between alpha-linolenic acid and cholesterol level. Salem et al. [28] proposed that docosahexanoic acid (DHA) controls the level of cholesterol as well as the composition and function of the neuronal membrane. Another approach [unpubl. data] suggests that the differential effects of omega–6 or omega–3 on the cholesterol level, depends on the activity of PUFA on reduced LDL-receptor activity. A negative correlation was found between membrane cholesterol level and improvement in learning capacity. A number of studies provide support for reducing neuronal membrane cholesterol by dietary supplementation of an omega–6/omega–3 compound in a ratio of 4:1 [29]. Such correlation was not found with other ratios. It is possible that this specific ratio (4:1) optimizes uptake of PUFA into the brain and promotes fatty acid incorporation into the neuronal membranes, while displacing cholesterol out of the membrane. The issue of the cholesterol neuronal membrane level is very important, as the level of cholesterol (and cholesterol metabolites) in the aging and in the Alzheimer's patient's brain is very high.

Omega–3 Deficiency

The method of inducing omega–3 deficiency via diet is a powerful tool to investigate the role of omega–3 in various brain functions. While most studies in this area involved the omega–3 deficiency issue, by definition, the ratio of omega–6 and omega–3 in experimental diets was different from the ratio in normal or balanced diets. Studies have shown that omega–3-deficient rats (mostly the 3rd generation with deficiency) exhibited poor learning and memory performances in a variety of tests, such as Morris Water Maze [30, 31], and olfactory-based learning and memory tasks, mainly in complex (vs. simple) learning [32, 33]. In addition, sensory deficits were evident in those rats, such as visual problems [34, 35]. One of Salem's studies [28] is of specific interest in this aspect; his omega–3-deficient rats showed very poor performance in spatial tasks and in olfactory-cued reversal learning tasks. However, he did not find any difference in the hippocampus gross morphology. Several hypotheses can be offered to explain the finding of poor learning. Omega–3 deficiency induces a significant decrease in the neuron size in the hippocampus, hypothalamus and cortex [36] – brain areas that mediate spatial and serial learning. In addition, omega–3 deficiency induces a significant reduction in cerebral catecholamines [37], in glucose transport capacity and glucose utilization in the brain [38], in the cyclic AMP level in the hippocampus [39], and in brain phospholipid synthesis capacity in the brain and in hypothalamus [40, 41]. Each one of those changes (in the levels of catecholamines, glucose, cAMP and phospholipids) can induce learning deficit.

The above-mentioned studies demonstrate two points; firstly, the essentiality of omega–3 fatty acids to the structure and normal function of the brain. Secondly, they demonstrate the importance of the ratio. It is impossible to induce omega–3 deficiency without offsetting the ratio between omega–6 and omega–3 in the diet. Though the authors did not specifically discuss the ratio of their control diet, our own calculations of the dietary information in the above-mentioned studies showed that they in fact used the ratio of omega–6/omega–3 of 4:1–5:1.

Early Development

Most studies on omega–3 deficiency singled the early development periods as an important, and almost 'critical' period for brain development.

Studies stress the importance of the influence of the fatty acids profile in mothers' milk on brain maturation. Jumpsen et al. [42, 43] showed that even small changes in the ratio of omega–6 to omega–3 in the diet, during neuronal and glial cell development, have significant effects on the development. He showed that a ratio of 4:1 was the optimal ratio for the development of the frontal cortex, hippocampus, cerebellum and glial cell number in developing rats. Small changes in the ratio, such as 6:1, impaired the rate of development.

Though the discussion whether the addition of long chain PUFA (LCPUFA) to baby formula is recommended is outside of the scope of this chapter, it seems that the importance of the level of PUFA and the omega–6/omega–3 ratio in the diet of the infant, in this sensitive development period, is emphasized by a great number of studies [44, 45, 23].

Learning and Memory

The above discussion demonstrated that various fatty acids serve different roles in the nervous system and in the body and it has been suggested that the nervous system has an absolute molecular species requirement for proper function. Studies in our laboratory confirm this finding, and even suggest an added qualifying requirement, viz. the need for a proper ratio between the essential fatty acids. Many studies examine the effects of various fatty acids on learning and memory, but very few examine the ratio between various PUFA. We experimentally tested our hypothesis that the ratio of omega–6 and omega–3 may be a key factor in modulating behavioral and neuropharmacological effects of polyunsaturated fatty acids. Therefore, we attempted to identify the optimal ratio. To avoid the variations that occur in the composition of fatty acids in commercially prepared oils, and to exclude the possible confounding effects of other fatty acids or lipid mixtures, we used highly purified linoleic and alpha-linolenic acids. We tested a wide range of ratios of linoleic/alpha-linolenic acid (3:1, 3.5:1, 4:1, 4.5:1, 5:1, 5.5:1, 6:1 (vol/vol)), which were administered as dietary supplements. All animal studies were conducted on rats, fed normal diets, as recommended by the American Institute of Nutrition (AIN). We found that a mixture of linoleic (omega–6) and alpha-linolenic acids (omega–3) with a ratio of 4:1 was the most effective in improving learning performance (as assessed by the Morris Water Maze, and passive avoidance), elevating pain threshold, improving sleep, and improving thermoregulation [46]. This ratio was also able to correct learning deficits induced by the neurotoxins AF64A and 5,7-dihydroxytryptamine [47], treatments that decrease the acetylcholine and serotonin brain levels. Similarly, this ratio overcame learning deficit induced by 6-OH-DA (e.g. reduction in brain dopamine level) [48]. Treatment with a single fatty acid was less successful [49, 50].

EFA, Aging and Alzheimer's Disease

Aging is a special period during development. The aging brain is different in many aspects from the adult brain. Among the many brain changes (e.g. decrease in the level of most neurotransmitters and hormones and an increase in cholesterol in the neuronal membrane) is that the level and the ratio of EFA is modified. PUFAs are major molecules responsible for regulating cellular differentiation and apoptosis [51]. Most of the studies on aging report a significant decrease in the level and turnover of PUFA [52–55]. This major change is a significant decrease in omega–3 fatty acids, such as α-linolenic and DHA [56]. The magnitude of the decrease in the ratio is not uniform in all brain areas. While the decrease is significant in the cortex, striatum and hypothalamus, the most profound decrease was found in the hippocampus [57]. During aging, there is a significant change in the transition temperature of the lipids, a change which is more profound in Alzheimer's patients [58]. This change causes the membrane to be more rigid. The most studied fatty acids, in this respect, are DHA (docosahexanoic, omega–3) and AA (arachidonic, omega–6). While the level of both fatty acids is very low in the neuronal membrane of the aged hippocampus in rats, treatment with omega–3 fatty acids improves the membrane status [59, 60]. Basically, there are two ways to explain the low level of PUFA in the aging brain, viz. the low rate of transport of PUFA from the blood into the brain, and the impaired biochemical machinery that normally is expected to incorporate and elongate the fatty acids. These two alternatives are directly related to their respective parent issues: the problem of the blood brain barrier and the dynamics of FA brain metabolism.

The brain of an Alzheimer's patient undergoes more severe changes than the brain of a healthy elderly person. Among the major changes, that are relevant to our issue, is (1) the decrease in the neurotransmitter acetylcholine in the brain (and in particular in the hippocampus), and (2) the major double change in the brain lipids, whereof one is the significant increase in cholesterol level in the neuronal membrane, accompanied by a decrease in total PUFA level. And the other is the change in the omega–6 and omega–3 ratio. The level of omega–3 fatty acids (mainly DHA) is severely reduced [61]. Those changes have direct effect on the membrane fluidity index, causing the membrane to become more rigid and eventually to malfunction.

Alzheimer's disease is a progressive and degenerative age-related dementia. Among the major symptoms are: short- and long-term memory loss, impairment of speech and language, decline of abstract reasoning, and mood change. The hallmark sign of Alzheimer's disorder is the loss of spatial orientation. Most researchers agree that the hippocampus is responsible for this function, and indeed postmortem studies showed shrinkage of the hippocampus in

Alzheimer's patients. The etiology of this disorder is not known, but many of the theories have been summarized in [62]. Our preliminary studies show that administration of a mixture of linoleic and alpha-linolenic acids, in a ratio of 4:1, improves the Mini Mental State Examination (MMSE) and quality of life test scores of Alzheimer's patients [62]. Treatments with other ratios did not improve the Alzheimer's patients' condition. Administrations of a single fatty acid, i.e. DHA, did not improve the Alzheimer's condition by much [63, 64]. These results reflect similar results that were obtained in animal experimental models of Alzheimer's.

Seizure

The relationship between lipids and fatty acid metabolism on the one hand, and seizures on the other, has been previously described [65, 66]. The general finding shows a gross disturbance in the fatty acid metabolisms [67–72]. One of the effects of a seizure is the transient disruption of the blood-brain barrier structure and functions [73, 74]. A well-known application of fatty acids in the diet for the treatment of epilepsy is represented by the ketogenic diet for children with refractory seizures [75, 76]. The promise of therapeutic effects that may be realized from ketogenic diets continues to be reaffirmed by many clinical investigators [77, 78].

The possible mode of action to account for the involvement of brain lipids in seizures was recently summarized [65]: Lipids are important constituents of the neuronal membrane and changes in the fatty acid profile may alter membrane functions.

1. Essential fatty acids and phospholipids may offset the deleterious effects of substances that induce seizures, such as iron, that have been shown to increase lipid peroxidation.
2. Essential fatty acids and phospholipids may offer stability in membrane fluidity that may otherwise be associated with seizures.
3. Essential fatty acids and phospholipids may control the alteration in neuronal membrane phospholipid metabolism that may result from the high prevalence of excitatory amino acid receptors in the epileptic focus.
4. A genetic link may exist between epilepsy and PUFA deficit [79], and a mixture of DHA and EPA may provide some measure of correction.
5. Essential fatty acids may serve as neuroprotectors in the brain, similar to effects observed in the heart, as shown in recent studies where alpha-linolenic acid (but not palmitic acid) was found to protect against ischemic-induced neuronal death, and to prevent kainic-induced seizures and its associated neuronal death [80, 81].

Apart from the interest in PUFA as a stabilizing agent for the neuronal membrane in seizure, is a growing interest in the use of the ketogenic diet in epileptic children. This diet is high-fat and low-carbohydrate, and is used to control intractable seizures in children. The abandoned ketogenic diet was very popular in the past and is currently being re-examined [82–85].

Multiple Sclerosis

Multiple sclerosis (MS) is characterized by active degradation of the central nervous system myelin, with clinical symptoms depending on the brain areas that are undergoing the demyelination. The etiology of MS is unknown; however, one of the major symptoms associated with MS is the deterioration of cognitive functions [86]. While an ideal animal model of MS unfortunately is unavailable, experimental allergic encephalomyelitis (EAE) is considered to be the best available substitute [87].

Relationships between MS disease and lipids and fatty acids have been proposed in the past [88, 89], with changes in lipid metabolism reported for MS patients [90, 91]. In addition, changes in the level of cholesterol in the brain of MS patients have been described [92].

Studies show that administration of a mixture of 4:1 omega–6 to omega–3 fatty acids, exerts beneficial effects in rats given a diluted dose of the EAE toxin. The EAE rats showed learning and motor deficits as well as major changes in the fatty acids profile and the cholesterol level in frontal cortex synaptosomes. This treatment was, to a significant degree, able to rehabilitate the changes induced by EAE, though not to completely reverse the deficits to the level of normal control. None of the other PUFA ratios were as effective as the ratio of 4:1 [93].

EFA and Sleep

Sleep quality is a major problem in the modern society. Vast numbers of 'healthy people' complain about the quality of their sleep. One of the major complaints is that sleep does not refresh them enough. In addition, many disease states are associated with objective or subjective sleep disturbances. The presumed neurochemical basis for the relationships between EFA and the different sleep stages was recently reviewed [11, 94].

We already showed that the particular EFA ratio of 4:1, when given to Alzheimer's patients, significantly reduced their complaints about sleep problems, and the quality of their sleep indeed improved [62].

Table 1. Effects of 4:1 ratio on rat sleep profile

	Before	After
Sleep quality	0.7 ± 0.3	0.5 ± 0.2*
Sleep latency	1.3 ± 0.4	0.7 ± 0.5**
Sleep duration	1.2 ± 0.3	0.6 ± 0.4**
Sleep efficiency	1.3 ± 0.4	0.7 ± 0.3**
Sleep disturbance	0.9 ± 0.4	0.4 ± 0.3**
Sleep medications	0.4 ± 0.2	0.3 ± 0.2 NS
Daytime dysfunction	1.4 ± 0.6	0.6 ± 0.3**
Sleep index total	7.2 ± 1.6	3.8 ± 1.8**

The numbers in each cell represent the mean and standard deviations of the score in each category. $*p < 0.05$; $**p < 0.01$.

In addition to the above, we have more data that has not yet been published. The new data includes three separate studies. In all the studies, a wide range of EFA ratios were tested, and in all the studies, the ratio of 4:1 was shown to be the optimal ratio. Two human studies were also performed:

(A) In an open trial, the 4:1 ratio was administered for 1 month (48 subjects, aged 24–46, 55% males and 45% females). The results showed improvement in the subjective feeling about sleep (as measured by interview). Only 3 subjects (out of the 48 subjects) said that their sleep was not improved. No other ratio had this high rate of success.

(B) 48 students (age: 21–27 years, 24 males and 24 females) were included in the study. All subjects were healthy, with no history of depression or sleep disturbances. In addition to the medical examination, each subject answered the Hebrew version of the sleep index (Pittsburgh Sleep Quality Index) before entering the study as well as on the 28th day of the study. The sleep index is intended to measure sleep quality and to identify good and bad sleepers. This index does not provide clinical diagnosis.

The Hebrew sleep index (Bar Ilan University addition, 2001) has 21 questions, examining seven subscales of sleep (three questions for each subscale). The subscales are: sleep quality; sleep latency; sleep duration; sleep efficiency; sleep disturbance; sleep medication; daytime dysfunction. The total score of the sleep index is between 0 and 21. The higher scores indicate poorer sleep. The researchers claim that a global score of above 5 may indicate that the subject has severe difficulties in two areas or moderate difficulties in three areas.

Table 1 shows the results of the study both as sleep index total scores and in each subscale. The total sleep index score decreases from 7.2 at the

Table 2. Effects of 4:1 ratio on rat sleep profile

	Before (n = 36)	Control no treatment (n = 12)	Control saline (n =12)	1:4 ratio (n = 12)
Wake	740.5 ± 28	740.9 ± 35	745.2 ± 29	770.4 ± 39*
Non-REM sleep	565.5 ± 22	584.9 ± 30	595 ± 42	540.9 ± 40*
REM sleep	100.7 ± 9	90.4 ± 12	102.7 ± 12	128.7 ± 14*
Motor activity 24 h	1,450 ± 100	1,528 ± 110	1,349 ± 136	1,772 ± 98*

The results of sleep profile are presented here as means in seconds. The data for motor activity are presented here as the means and standard deviation of total motor movements for a 24-hour period. *$p < 0.05$.

beginning of the study to 3.8 after 28 days ($p < 0.001$). In all the subscales, except one, statistical significant differences ($p < 0.001$) were found. Only the subscale of 'sleep medication' was not affected in this study. The use of sleep medications in this age group is rare, and the baseline was very low.

In conclusion, the 4:1 ratio showed beneficial effects in this group of students. This is a group which is generally highly stressed and the general comment was that the 4:1 ratio helped them to study more effectively.

In order to investigate the effects of the 4:1 ratio on sleep parameters in rats, a group of Sprague-Dawley male (about 200 g body weight) rats (n = 36) were used. EEG electrodes were fixed to the rats' heads. All materials and methods are described in the paper by Conrad et al. [95]. The cage of each rat was on an activity meter. The original group of 36 rats was divided randomly into three groups: (1) no treatment for 4 weeks; (2) a daily i.p. injection of saline for 4 weeks, and (3) a daily injection of 40 mg/kg 4:1 ratio for 4 weeks. Measurements of EEG profile and motor activity were done on days 0 and 28. The results are presented in table 2.

The results show that the 4:1 ratio treated rats improved their sleep profile. They were awake for a longer period of time, the REM sleep periods were longer, and they had shorter non-REM periods. The total motor activity level was higher in the 4:1 ratio treated group. The difference between the 4:1 ratio group at day 28 and the other groups is statistically significant ($p < 0.05$).

The combined results of human and rat studies clearly indicate that the 4:1 ratio only possesses beneficial effects on sleep quality and therefore on daytime performance.

Stress, Cortisol and Learning

The importance of the differentiation among the various types of fatty acids may be appreciated by noting their effects on immunological and endocrinological factors. For example, omega–3 fatty acids suppress the synthesis of interleukin-1 and 6 and enhance the synthesis of interleukin-2, while omega–6 fatty acids have the opposite effect. It should be recalled that both interleukin-6 and interleukin-1 (and to a lesser degree interleukin-2) promote the corticotropin-releasing factor (CRF) release via arachidonic acid. However, CRF inhibits the stimulating effect of interleukin-1 on the prostaglandin synthesis.

Cortisol exerts powerful effects on all body tissues. It increases the level of glucose in the blood, stimulates the breakdown of proteins into amino acids, inhibits the uptake of glucose by muscle tissues (except in the brain) and regulates the response of the cardiovascular system to persistent high blood pressure. All of these actions constitute the 'fight or flight' response, which helps the organism to cope with stress situations. Recent studies, however, indicate that cortisol may have some damaging effects, including deterioration of learning and memory. Human studies on normal, aged, depressed, Cushing's syndrome patients, as well as mentally ill patients, have demonstrated a strong negative correlation between cortisol levels and learning and memory in a wide range of cognitive tasks. In rats, cortisol induces deterioration in spatial task performance as measured by the Morris Water Maze (MWM) test. These negative effects may be explained by the fact that cortisol interferes with physiological mechanisms crucial to the structure, and function of the hippocampus. For example, stress is known to cause atrophy of the hippocampal dendrites, damage to the pyramidal neurons, and to interfere with synaptic activity. It is most likely that this morphological and functional hippocampal damage results from high levels of cortisol.

Recently we demonstrated that a specific mixture of free essential fatty acids [linoleic ($18:2\omega6$) and alpha-linolenic ($18:3\omega3$)] is able to reduce the levels of cholesterol in brain neuronal membranes [96, 20].

Hippocampal functions, which include spatial learning abilities, can be assessed through the MWM. This popular test is used to evaluate potential drugs for Alzheimer's disorder, since Alzheimer's patients exhibit great difficulties in spatial orientation. Independent of hippocampal effects, hypothermia was also shown to impair learning, as evaluated by using various tests, including the MWM performance test, which is specially meant for spatial learning.

Further interest in the relationships between cortisol and learning arose when recent findings showed an increase in the level of cortisol in Alzheimer's patients, who were also shown to have elevated levels of interleukin-6 (IL-6). It should be noted that IL-6 receptors were found in the adrenal cortex, and that the level of cortisol is raised by IL-6, which in turn is increased by general stress and cold.

Our study [97] showed that a mixture of linoleic and alpha-linolenic acids, administered for 3 weeks prior to injection of cortisol (10 mg/kg), or prior to immersion of rats in a 10°C saline bath, blocked the elevation of cortisol and cholesterol blood levels. In addition, this treatment protected the rats from the spatial learning deficits that usually accompany the stressful conditions in the Morris Water Maze. Moreover, a recent study showed that certain anti epileptic drugs induce an increase in the cortisol level. The PUFA mixture at a 4:1 ratio can reduce the elevated cortisol level and has anti convulsant effects [98]. Only this ratio has the effect of decreasing elevated cortisol levels.

Conclusions

This review related mainly to linoleic and alpha-linolenic acids. The ratio between omega–6 and omega–3 can also be maintained by using longer chain fatty acids, such as AA and DHA. However, very few studies have been carried out on the balance between the LCPUFA balance or ratio and brain function. The few studies, that in fact did examine this area, were recently summarized [99, 100], and demonstrated the importance of the ratio between omega–6 and omega–3.

It might very well be that the required ratio of omega–6 and omega–3 may differ when used for different tissues or functions. One can understand that a ratio of 1:1 is the optimal ratio for preventing cardiovascular diseases, and another ratio would be optimal for cancer prevention. We are merely suggesting that a ratio of 4:1 is the optimal ratio for brain-mediated functions. The question is; how can it be that PUFA is of help to organisms that are only capable of obtaining it from the diet? Our hypothesis is that omega–6 and omega–3, in a ratio of 4:1, act within the neuronal membrane and improves the membrane fluidity index, which is the key to all neuronal activity. Other researchers have also recommended the ratio of 4:1. The results of those studies were earlier summarized by Yehuda and Carasso [46], and again more recently by Horrocks and Yeo [101]. We have difficulties explaining why this particular ratio is best. One possibility is that the preferred ratio for omega–6 and omega–3 PUFA depends on the competition of the same enzymes for desaturation and elongation. Another possibility is that PUFA, in this ratio, are able to create micella, which protects them. Whatever the biochemical basis could be, the results showed that the 4:1 ratio has protective and stabilizing effects on the neuronal membrane.

Acknowledgements

I would like to thank Dr. Sharon Rabinovitz-Shenkar and Ms. Ingrid Muller for their very helpful comments on this manuscript. Furthermore, I would like to thank the Rose K. Ginsburg

Chair for Research into Alzheimer's disease and the William Center for Alzheimer's Research for continued support.

References

1   Simopoulos AP: Evolutionary aspects of omega–3 fatty acids in the food supply. Prostaglandins Leukot Essent Fatty Acids 1999;60:421–429.
2   Feller SE, Gawrisch K, MacKerell AD Jr: Polyunsaturated fatty acids in lipid bilayers: Intrinsic and environmental contributions to their unique physical properties. J Am Chem Soc 2002;124:318–326.
3   Yehuda S, Rabinovitz S, Mostofsky DI: PUFA: Mediators for the Nervous, endocrine, and Immune System; in Mostofsky DI, Yehuda S, Salem N (eds): Fatty Acids: Physiological and Behavioral Functions. New York, Humana Press, 2001, pp 403–420.
4   Rapoport SI: In vivo fatty acid incorporation into brain phospholipids in relation to plasma availability, signal transduction and membrane remodeling. J Mol Neurosci 2001;16:243–261.
5   Edmond J: Essential polyunsaturated fatty acids and the barrier to the brain. J Mol Neurosci 2001;16:181–193.
6   de la Torre JC, Mussivand T: Can disturbed brain microcirculation cause Alzheimer's disease? Neurol Res 1993;15:146–153.
7   Ginsberg L, Xeureb JH, Gershfeld NL: Membrane instability plasmalogen content and Alzheimer's disease. J Neurochem 1998;70:2533–2538.
8   Strosznajder J, Samochocki M, Duran M: Aging diminishes serotonin-stimulated arachidonic acid uptake and cholinergic receptor-activated acid release in rat brain cortex membrane. J Neurochem 1994;62:1048–1054.
9   Terracina L, Brunetti M, Avellini L, de Medio GE, Trovarelli G, Gaiti A: Linoleic acid metabolism in brain cortex of aged rats. Ital J Biochem 1992;41:225–235.
10 Su HM, Huang MC, Saad NM, Nathanielsz PW, Brenna JT: Fetal baboons convert 18:3n-3 to 22:6n-3 in vivo: A stable isotope tracer study. J Lipid Res 2001;42:581–586.
11 Yehuda S, Rabinovitz S, Carasso RL, Mostofsky DI: Fatty acids and brain peptides. Peptides 1998; 19:407–419.
12 Zimmer L, Delpal S, Guilloteau D, Aioun J, Durand G: Chronic n-3 polyunsaturated fatty acid deficiency alters dopamine vesicle density in the rat frontal cortex. Neurosci Lett 2000;284:25–28.
13 Zimmer L, Vancassel S, Cantagrel S, Breton P, Delamanche S, Guilloteau D, Durand G, Chalon S: The dopamine mesocorticolimbic pathway is affected by deficiency in n-3 polyunsaturated fatty acids. Am J Clin Nutr 2002;75:662–667.
14 Kodas E, Vancassel S, Lejeune B, Guilloteau D, Chalon S: Reversibility of n-3 fatty acid deficiency-induced changes in dopaminergic neurotransmission in rats: Critical role of developmental stage. J Lipid Res 2002;43:1209–1219.
15 Chalon S, Delion-Vancassel S, Belzung C, Guilloteau D, Lequisquet AM, Besnard JC, Durand G: Dietary fish oil effects monoaminergic neurotransmission and behavior in rats. J Nutr 1998;128: 2512–2519.
16 Acar N, Chardigny JM, Darbois M, Pasquis B, Sebedio JL: Modification of the dopaminergic neurotransmitters in striatum, frontal cortex and hippocampus of rats fed for 21 months with trans isomers of alpha-linolenic acid. Neurosci Res 2003;45:375–382.
17 Farkas E, de Wilde MC, Kiliaan A, Meijer J, Keijser JN, Luiten PGM: Dietary long chain PUFAs differentially effect hippocampal muscarinic 1 and serotonergic 1A receptors in experimental cerebral hypoperfusion. Brain Res 2002;954:32–41.
18 Yehuda S, Rabinovitz S, Mostofsky DI: Essential fatty acids are mediators of brain biochemistry and cognitive functions. J Neurosci Res 1999;15:565–570.
19 Yehuda S, Rabinovitz S, Carasso RL, Mostofsky DT: The Role of PUFA in restoring the aging neuronal membrane. Neurobiol Aging 2002;23:843–853.
20 Yehuda S, Rabinovitz S, Mostofsky DI: Modulation of learning and neuronal membrane composition in the rat by essential fatty acids preparation: Time course analysis. Neurochem Res 1998; 23:631–638.

21 Auestad N: Infant nutrition – brain development – disease in later life. Dev Neurosci 2000;22:472–473.

22 Salvati S, Attorri L, Avellino C, Di Biase A, Sanchez M: Diet, lipids and brain development. Dev Neurosci 2000;22:481–487.

23 Stockard JE, Saste MD, Benford VJ, Barness L, Auestad N, Carver JD: Effect of docosahexaenoic acid content of maternal diet on auditory brainstem conduction times in rat pups. Dev Neurosci 2000;22:494–499.

24 Youdim MBH, Yehuda S: The neurochemical basis of cognitive deficits induced by brain iron deficiency: Involvement of dopamine-opiate system. Cell Molec Biol 2000;46:491–500.

25 Ando S, Tanaka Y, Toyoda Y, Kon K: Turnover of myelin lipids in aging brain. Neurochem Res 2003;28:5–13.

26 Horrocks LA, Harder HW: Fatty acids and cholesterol; in Lajtha A (ed): Handbook of Neurochemistry. Plenum, New York, 1983, pp 1–16.

27 Bourre JM, Dumont O, Piciotti M, Clement M, Chaudiere J, Bonneil M, et al: Essentiality of w3 fatty acids for brain structure and function. World Rev Nutr. Basel, Karger, 1991, vol 66, pp 103–117.

28 Salem N, Moriguchi T, Greiner RS, McBride K, Ahmad A, Catalan JN, Slotnick B: Alterations in brain function after loss of docosahexaenoate due to dietary restriction of n-3 fatty acids. J Mol Neurosci 2001;16:299–307.

29 Yehuda S, Rabinovitz S, Mostofsky DI: Effects of essential fatty acids preparation (SR-3) on brain biochemistry and on behavioral and cognitive functions; in Yehuda S, Mostofsky DI (eds): Handbook of Essential Fatty Acids Biology: Biochemistry Physiology and Behavioral Neurobiology. New York, Humana Press, 1997, pp 427–452.

30 Moriguchi T, Greiner RS, Salem N: Behavioral deficits associated with dietary induction of decreased brain docosahexaenoic acid concentration. J Neurochem 2000;75:2563–2573.

31 Wainwright PE: Dietary essential fatty acids and brain function: A developmental perspective on mechanisms. Proc Nutr Soc 2002;61:61–69.

32 Greiner RS, Moriguchi T, Slotnick BM, Hutton A, Salem N: Olfactory discrimination deficits in n-3 acid-deficient rats. Physiol Behav 2001;72:379–385.

33 Catalan J, Moriguchi T, Slotnick B, Murthy M, Greiner RS, Salem N: Cognitive deficits in docosahexaenoic acid-deficient rats. Behav Neurosci 2002;116:1022–1031.

34 Jeffrey BG, Mitchell DC, Gibson RA, Neuringer M: n-3 fatty acid deficiency alters recovery of the rod photoresponse in rhesus monkeys. Invest Ophthalmol Vis Sci 2002;43:2806–2814.

35 Jeffrey BG, Mitchell DC, Hibbeln JR, Gibson RA, Chedester AL, Salem N: Visual acuity and retinal function in infant monkeys fed long-chain PUFA. Lipids 2002;37:839–848.

36 Ahmad A, Murthy M, Greiner RS, Moriguchi T, Salem N: A decrease in cell size accompanies a loss of docosahexaenoate in the rat hippocampus. Nutr Neurosci 2002;5:103–113.

37 Takeuchi T, Fukumoto Y, Harada E: Influence of a dietary n-3 fatty acid deficiency on the cerebral catecholamine contents, EEG and learning ability in rat. Behav Brain Res 2002;131:193–203.

38 Ximenes da Silva A, Lavialle F, Gendrot G, Guesnet P, Alessandri JM, Lavialle M: Glucose transport and utilization are altered in the brain of rats deficient in n-3 polyunsaturated fatty acids. J Neurochem 2002;81:1328–1337.

39 Nanjo A, Kanazawa A, Sato K, Banno F, Fujimoto K: Depletion of dietary n-3 fatty acid affects the level of cyclic AMP in rat hippocampus. J Nutr Sci Vitaminol 1999;45:633–641.

40 Gazzah N, Gharib A, Croset M, Bobillier P, Lagarde M, Sarda N: Decrease of brain phospholipid synthesis in free-moving n-3 fatty acid deficient rats. J Neurochem 1995;64:908–918.

41 Murthy M, Hamilton J, Greiner RS, Moriguchi T, Salem N, Kim HY: Differential effects of n-3 fatty acid deficiency on phospholipid molecular species composition in the rat hippocampus. J Lipid Res 2002;43:611–617.

42 Jumpsen J, Lien EL, Goh YK, Clandinin MT: Small changes of dietary (n-6) and (n-3)/ fatty acid content ratio alter phosphatidylethanolamine and phosphatidylcholine fatty acid composition during development of neuronal and glial cells in rats. J Nutr 1997;127:724–731.

43 Jumpsen JA, Lien EL, Goh YK, Clandinin MT: During neuronal and glial cell development diet n-6 to n-3 fatty acid ratio alters the fatty acid composition of phosphatidylinositol and phosphatidylserine. Biochim Biophys Acta 1997;1347:40–50.

44   Wainwright PE, Xing HC, Mutsaers L, McCutcheon D, Kyle D: Arachidonic acid offsets the effects on mouse brain and behavior of a diet with a low (n-6):(n-3) ratio and very high levels of docosahexaenoic acid. J Nutr 1997;127:184–193.

45   Xiang M, Alfven G, Blennow M, Trygg M, Zetterstrom R: Long-chain polyunsaturated fatty acids in human milk and brain growth during early infancy. Acta Paediatr 2000;89:142–147.

46   Yehuda S, Carasso RL: Modulation of learning, pain thresholds, and thermoregulation in the rat by preparations of free purified r-linolenic and linoleic acids: Determination of optimal n-3 to omega–6 ratio. Proc Natl Acad Sci USA 1993;90:10345–10349.

47   Yehuda S, Carasso RL, Mostofsky DI: Essential fatty acid preparation (1:4 ratio) rehabilitates learning deficits induced by AF64A and 5,7-DHT. NeuroReport 1995;6:511–515.

48   Yehuda S, Rabinovitz S, Mostofsky DI: Polyunsaturated fatty acids mixture treatment prevents deleterious effects of Ro4–1284. Eur J Pharmacol, 1999;365:27–34.

49   Ikemoto A, Ohishi M, Sato Y, Hata N, Misawa Y, Fujii Y, Okuyama H: Reversibilityof n-3 fatty acid deficiency-induced alterations of learning behavior in the rat: Level of n-6 fatty acids as another critical factor. J Lipid Res 2001;42:1655–1663.

50   Umezawa M, Kogishi K, Tojo H, Yoshimura S, Seriu N, Ohta A, Takeda T, Hosokawa M: High-linoleate and high-alpha-linolenate diets affect learning ability and natural behavior in SAMR1 mice. J Nutr 1999;129:431–437.

51   Sawazaki S, Hamazaki T, Yazawa K, Kobayashi M: The effect of docosahexaenoic acid on plasma catecholamine concentrations and glucose tolerance during long-lasting psychological stress: A double blind placebo-controlled study. J Nutr Neurosci Vitaminol 1999;45:655–665.

52   Favreliere S, Stadelman-Ingrand S, Huguet F, De Javel D, Piriou A, Tallineau C, et al: Age-related changes in ethanolamine glycerophospholipid fatty acid levels in rat frontal cortex and hippocampus. Neurobiol Aging 2000;21:653–660.

53   Regev R, Assaraf YG, Eytan GD: Membrane fluidization by ether other anesthetics, and certain agents abolishes P-glycoprotein ATPase activity and modulates efflux from multidrug-resistant cells. Eur J Biochem 1999;258:18–24.

54   Vreugdenhil M, Bruehl C, Voskuyl RA, Kang JX, Leaf A, Wadman WJ: Polyunsaturated fatty acids modulate sodium and calcium currents in CA1 neurons. Proc Natl Acad Sci USA 1996;93: 12559–12563.

55   Zaidi A, Michaelis ML: Effects of reactive oxygen species on brain synapticplasma membrane Ca(2+)-ATPase. Free Rad Biol Med 1999;27:810–821.

56   Favreliere S, Perault MC, Huguet F, De Javel D, Bertrand N, Piriou A, Durand G: DHA-enriched phospholipid diets modulate age-related alterations in rat hippocampus. Neurobiol Aging 2003; 24:233–243.

57   Ulmann L, Mimouni V, Roux S, Porsolt R, Poisson JP: Brain and hippocampus fatty acid composition in phospholipid classes of age-relative cognitive deficit rats. Prostaglandins Leukot Essent Fatty Acids 2001;64:189–195.

58   Giorgi PL, Biraghi M, Kantar A: Effect of desmopressin on rat brain synaptosomal membrane: A pilot study. Curr Therap Res 1998;59:172–178.

59   McGahon BM, Murray CA, Horrobin DF, Lynch MA: Age-related changes in oxidative mechanisms and LTP are reversed by dietary manipulation. Neurobiol Aging 1999;20:643–653.

60   Meehan E, Beauge F, Choquart D, Laonard BE: Influence of an n-6 polyunsaturated fatty acid-enriched diet on the development of tolerance during chronic ethanol administration in rats. Alcohol Clin Exp Res 1995;1:1441–1446.

61   Conquer JA, Tierney MC, Zecevic J, Bettger WJ, Fisher RH: Fatty acid analysis of blood plasma of patients with Alzheimer's disease, other types of dementia, and cognitive impairment. Lipids 2000;35:1305–1312.

62   Yehuda S, Rabinovitz S, Carasso RL, Mostofsky DI: Essential fatty acids preparation (1:4 ratio) improved Alzheimer's patients quality of life. Inter J Neurosci 1996;87:141–149.

63   Hashimoto M, Hossain S, Shimada T, Sugioka K, Yamasaki H, Fujii Y, Ishibashi Y, Oka JI, Shido O: Docosahexaenoic acid provides protection from impairment of learning ability in Alzheimer's disease model rats. J Neurochem 2002;81:1084–1091.

64   Das UN: Beneficial effect(s) of n-3 fatty acids in cardiovascular diseases: But, why and how? Prostaglandins Leukot Essent Fatty Acids 2000;63:351–362.

65 Yehuda S, Carasso RL, Mostofsky DI: Essential fatty acid preparation (1:4 ratio) raises the seizure threshold in rats. Eur J Pharmacol 1994;254:193–198.

66 Lauritzen L, Hansen HS, Jorgensen MH, Michaelsen KF: The essentiality of long chain n-3 fatty acids in relation to development and function of the brain and retina. Prog Lipid Res 2001;40:1–94.

67 Bazan NG: The neuromessenger platelet-activating factor in plasticity neurodegeneration. Prog Brain Res 1986;118:281–291.

68 Pediconi MF, Rodriguez de Turco EB, Bazan NG: Reduced labeling of brain phosphatidylinositol, triacylglycerols, and diacylglycerols by [C]arachidonic acid after electroconvulsive shock: Potentiation of the effect by edrenergic drugs and comparison with palmitic acid labeling. Neurochem Res 1986;11:1–14.

69 Van Rooijen LA, Vadnal R, Dobard P, Bazan NG: Enhanced inositide turnover in brain during bicuculline-induced status epilepticus. Biochem Biophys Res Commun 1986;136:827–834.

70 Flynn CJ, Wecker L: Concomitant increases in the levels of choline and free fatty acids in rat brain: evidence supporting the seizure-induced hydrolysis of phosphatidylcholine. J Neurochem 1987;48:1178–1184.

71 Visioli F, Rodriguez de Turco EB, Kreisman NR, Bazan NG: Membrane lipid degration is related to interictal cortical activity in a series of seizures. Metab Brain Dis 1994;9:161–170.

72 Birkle DL: Regional and temporal variations in the accumulation of unesterified fatty acids and diacylglycerols in the rat brain during kainic acid induced limbic seizures. Brain Res 1993;613:115–122.

73 Cornford EM, Oldendorf WH: Epilepsy and the blood-brain barrier. Adv Neurol 1986;44:787–812.

74 Cervos-Navarro J, Kannuki S, Nakagawa Y: Blood-brain barrier (BBB). Review from morphological aspect. Histol Histopathol 1988;3:203–213.

75 Stafstrom CE, Bough KJ: The ketogenic diet for the treatment of epilepsy: A challenge for nutritional neuroscientists. Nutr Neurosci 2003;6:67–79.

76 Freeman JM, Vining EP, Pillas DJ, Pyzik PL, Casey JC, Kelly LM: The efficacy of the ketogenic diet-1998: A prospective evaluation of intervention in 150 children. Pediatrics 1998;102:1358–1363.

77 Ben-Menachem E: New antiepileptic drugs and non-pharmaceutical treatments. Curr Opin Neurol 2000;13:165–170.

78 Helmstaedter C, Kurthen: Memory and epilepsy: Characteristics, course and influence of drugs and surgery. Curr Opin Neurol 2001;14:211–216.

79 Søvik O, Mansson JE, Bjorke Monsen AL, Jellum E, Berge RK: Generalized peroxisomal disorder in male twins: Fatty acid composition of serum lipids and response to n-3 fatty acids. J Inherit Metab Dis 1998;21:662–670.

80 Xiao Y, Li JX: Polyunsaturated fatty acids modify mouse hippocampal neuronal excitability during excitotoxic or convulsant stimulation. Brain Res 1999;846:112–121.

81 Lauritzen I, Blondeau N, Heurteaux C, Widmann GR, Lazdunski M: Polyunsaturated fatty acids are potent neuroprotectors. EMBO J 2000;19:1784–1793.

82 Thavendiranathan P, Chow C, Cunnane S, Burnham WM: The effect of the 'classic' ketogenic diet on animal seizure models. Brain Res 2003;959:206–213.

83 Cunnane SC, Musa K, Ryan MA, Whiting S, Fraser DD: Potential role of polyunsaturates in seizure protection achieved with the ketogenic diet. Prostaglandins Leukot Essent Fatty Acids 2002;67:131–135.

84 Musa-Veloso K, Rarama E, Comeau F, Curtis R, Cunnane S: Epilepsy and the ketogenic diet: Assessment of ketosis in children using breath acetone. Pediatr Res 2002;52:443–448.

85 Klepper J, Leiendecker B, Bredahl R, Athanassopoulos S, Heinen F, Gertsen E, Flörcken A, Metz A, Voit T: Introduction of a ketogenic diet in young infants. J Inherit Metab Dis 2002; 25:449–460.

86 Ron AM, Feinstein A: Multiple sclerosis and the mind. J Neurol Neurosurg Psychiatry 1992;55:1–3.

87 Werkele H: Lymphocyte traffic to the brain; in Pardridge WM (ed); The Blood Brain Barrier. Raven Press, New York, 1993, pp 67–83.

88 Swank RL, Grimsgaard A: Multiple sclerosis: The lipid relationship. Am J Clin 1988;48:1387–1393.

89 Williams KA, Deber, CM: The structure and function of central nervous system myelin. Crit Rev Clin Lab Sci 1993;30:29–64.

90 Holman RT, Johnson SB, Kokmen E: Deficiencies of polyunsaturated fatty acids and replacement by nonessential fatty acids in plasma lipids in multiple sclerosis. Proc Natl Acad Sci USA 1989; 86:4720–4724.

91 Nightingale S, Woo, E, Smith AD, French JM, Gale MM, Sinclair HM, Bates D, Shaw DA: Red blood cell and adipose tissue fatty acids in mild inactive multiple sclerosis. Acta Neurol Scand 1990;82:43–50.

92 Nicholas, HJ, Taylor J: Central nervous system demyelinating diseases and increased release of cholesterol into the urinary system of rats. Lipids 1994;29:611–617.

93 Yehuda S, Rabinovitz S, Mostofsky DI, Huberman M, Carasso RL, Sredni B: Essential fatty acid preparation improves biochemical and cognitive functions in EAE rats. Eur J Pharmacol 1997; 328:23–29.

94 Yehuda S, Rabinovitz S, Mostofsky DI: Essential fatty acids and sleep: Mini review and hypothesis. Med Hypothesis 1998;50:139–145.

95 Conrad A, Bull DF, King MG, Husband AJ: The effects of lipopolysaccharide (LPS) on the fever response in rats at different ambient temperatures. Physiol Behav 1997;62:1197–1201.

96 Yehuda S, Brandys Y, Mostofsky DI, Blumenfeld A: Essential fatty acid preparation reduces cholesterol and fatty acids in rat cortex. Inter J Neurosci 1996;86:249–256.

97 Yehuda S, Rabinovitz S, Carasso RL, Mostofsky DI: Fatty acid mixture counters changes in cortisol, cholesterol and impair learning. Int J Neurosci 2000;101:73–87.

98 Rabinovitz S, Mostofsky DI, Yehuda S: Anticonvulsant efficiency, behavioral performance and cortisol level: A comparison of carbamazepine (CBZ) and a fatty acid compound (SR-3). Psychoneuroendocrinology 2003;in press.

99 Simopoulos AP: Human requirement for N-3 polyunsaturated fatty acids. Poult Sci 2000;79:961–970.

100 Youdim KA, Martin A, Joseph JA: Essential fatty acids and the brain: Possible health implications. Int J Dev Neurosci 2000;18:383–399.

101 Horrocks LA, Yeo YK: Health benefits of docosahexaenoic acid (DHA). Pharmacol Res 1999; 40:211–225.

Prof. Shlomo Yehuda, Psychopharmacology Laboratory
Department of Psychology, Bar Ilan University
Ramat Gan 52900 (Israel)
Tel. +972 3 5318583, Fax +972 3 5353327, E-Mail yehudas@mail.biu.ac.il

Simopoulos AP, Cleland LG (eds): Omega–6/Omega–3 Essential Fatty Acid Ratio:
The Scientific Evidence. World Rev Nutr Diet. Basel, Karger, 2003, vol 92, pp 57–73

....

Dietary Prevention of Coronary Heart Disease: Focus on Omega–6/Omega–3 Essential Fatty Acid Balance

Michel de Lorgeril, Patricia Salen

Laboratoire du Stress Cardiovasculaire et Pathologies Associées,
UFR de Médecine et Pharmacie, Grenoble, France

Alpha-linolenic acid, ALA or $18:3\omega3$, is one of the two essential fatty acids in humans. The other one is linoleic acid, LA or $18:2\omega6$. The term *essential* means that these fatty acids must be supplied in the diet because the body needs them but cannot synthesize them. Humans actually lack the enzymes to introduce double bonds at carbon atoms beyond carbon 9 in the fatty acid chain. LA and ALA obtained from the diet are the starting point for the synthesis of a variety of other unsaturated fatty acids. After ingestion, ALA is converted into very long-chain polyunsaturated fatty acids (PUFAs), i.e. readily to eicosapentanoic acid, EPA or $20:5\omega3$, and more slowly to docosahexanoic acid, DHA or $22:6\omega3$. Using the same pathways (the same enzymes) and in competition with ALA, LA is converted into arachidonic acid, AA or $20:4\omega6$, which is, in competition (again) with EPA, the starting point for the synthesis of eicosanoids and prostaglandins that are important mediators in many inflammatory diseases and in particular in cardiovascular diseases. Briefly, the prostaglandins, thromboxanes and leukotrienes derived from $20:5\omega3$ have different biological properties than do those derived from $20:4\omega6$, i.e. their global effects result in less vasoconstriction, platelet aggregation and leukocyte toxicity. Importantly, enzymes forming prostaglandin autacoids (COX-1 and COX-2) act faster with $20:4\omega6$ than $20:5\omega3$, which results in a considerable amplification of inflammation when the $20:4\omega6/20:5\omega3$ ratio is high [1, 2]. Thus, when the LA/ALA ratio decreases as a result of dietary changes, $20:5\omega3$ competes with $20:4\omega6$ for eicosanoid metabolism at the cyclooxygenase and lipoxygenase levels in platelets and leukocytes. As a result, the balance between metabolites stimulating platelets and leukocytes (and also having vasoconstrictive properties) and metabolites with opposing properties shifts towards those with antithrombotic, anti-inflammatory and vasodilative properties. A major consequence of ALA deficiency is that its chief synthetic end products, especially 22:6ω3, are not adequately produced. Because 22:6ω3 is a major component of the phospholipid membranes of the brain and retina, its deficiency in these organs leads to functional abnormalities [3, 4]. Phospholipids in the myocardium and the myocardial membrane are also rich in 22:6ω3. This is very important in case of ischemia, in particular for the ability of the ischemic or the postischemic myocardium not to develop arrhythmias [5]. Deficiency in omega–3 fatty acids is higher when the dietary supply of LA (found in corn and sunflower oils, for instance) is high at the same time, because of the competition between ALA and LA for their entry in the elongation and desaturation pathways leading to the synthesis of long-chain PUFAs and then of eicosanoids. Thus, a high ratio of omega–6 to omega–3 PUFAs in the diet tends to increase a deficiency in ALA [6]. The paradox of the competition between LA and ALA is that there is a huge difference in their blood concentrations. For instance, with people following a Western type of diet, the plasma ALA level is about 0.30% of total plasma fatty acids whereas the concentration of LA is about 30%. Thus, the ratio of LA to ALA in blood is about 100 to 1. Because the enzymes involved in the metabolism of LA and ALA (elongases and desaturases) prefer ALA to LA [7], a small change in dietary intake results in highly significant changes in the omega–6 to omega–3 ratios in both plasma and cell membranes [8].

The symptoms associated with a relative ALA deficiency have not been specifically outlined in the cardiovascular area to date. In fact, the potential effects of ALA on cardiovascular diseases were discovered when it was reported that populations with a high proportion of ALA in plasma lipids (the Greek and Japanese cohorts of the Seven Countries Study, for instance) are apparently protected from cardiovascular diseases [9], and when it was found that these low-risk populations consume foods rich in ALA [10, 11]. It was the merit of Simopoulos et al. [10] to show that many green leafy vegetables (such as purslane) largely consumed around the Mediterranean basin are a major source of ALA for the Cretan population at that period. The Cretan diet is also rich in antioxidants. This is a major point since because of its three double bonds, ALA is highly sensitive to oxidation and a high intake of ALA must be combined with a high intake of antioxidants to protect it from oxidation. The same authors also reported that eggs from range-fed Greek hens (which make a feast of purslane and other ALA-rich fresh green grass) are richer in ALA and other omega–3 fatty acids than eggs bought in US supermarkets which are, in turn, usually rich in LA [11]. The large difference in the fatty acid composition of the two types of eggs was indeed also due to the fatty acid composition of the industrial feedstuff given to US hens. This suggested that egg yolk might have been a considerable source of ALA and other omega–3 fatty acids for people living in the Mediterranean area, one of the regions of the world where the incidence of (and mortality from) coronary heart disease (CHD) is low. The point is important because this population usually does not consume large amounts of marine products rich in very long-chain omega–3 fatty acids.

Another important point to encourage the consumption of ALA and to reduce the intake of LA (with a significant decrease in the omega–6/omega–3 ratios) came from the observation that the lowest ex vivo platelet aggregation measured in humans in response to adenosine diphosphate, a possible indicator of the risk of acute CHD events, was recorded with a dietary LA to ALA ratio of about 4 to 1 [12, 13], i.e. much lower than that of the present Western diet and also lower than what many experts recommend at present. This pointed out the potential importance of ALA to prevent the thrombotic complications of CHD [14]. However, it remains that only randomised trials could bring definite information regarding causal relationships. The next section will provide some data regarding recent dietary trials.

The Lyon Diet Heart Study

The Lyon Diet Heart Study is a secondary prevention trial designed to test the hypothesis that a Mediterranean ALA-rich diet may improve the prognosis of patients having survived a first acute myocardial infarction [15]. The design, methods and results of the trial have been reported [15–17]. A striking protective effect of that Mediterranean diet was reported with a 50–70% reduction of the risk of recurrence after 4 years of follow-up [18]. Briefly, as regards lipids, the experimental Mediterranean diet tested in the trial supplied less than 30% of energy from fats and less than 8% of energy from saturated fats. Regarding essential fatty acids, the intake of LA was restricted to 4% of energy and the intake of ALA made up more than 0.6% of energy. In practical terms, the dietary instructions were detailed and customized to each patient [15–17] and can be summarized as: more bread, more cereals, more legumes and beans, more fresh vegetables and fruits, more fish, less meat (beef, lamb, pork) and delicatessen, which were to be replaced by poultry; no more butter and cream, to be replaced by an experimental canola oil-based margarine. This margarine was chemically comparable with olive oil but slightly enriched in LA and mostly in ALA, the two essential fatty acids. Finally, the oils recommended for salad and food preparation were exclusively olive and canola (erucid acid-free rapeseed oil) oils. The scientific rationale for that 'dietary fat strategy' has been discussed elsewhere [15–17]. Briefly, it was hypothesized that, because the lowest rates of cardiovascular diseases in the world were observed in populations

Table 1. Main characteristics of the diet in the two groups of the Lyon Diet Heart Study at the end of the trial [15–18] (% calories)

	Control	Experimental	p
Total calories	2,088 (490)	1,947 (468)	0.033
Total lipids	33.6 (7.80)	30.4 (7.00)	0.002
Saturated fats	11.7 (3.90)	8.0 (3.70)	0.0001
Polyunsaturated fats	6.10 (2.90)	4.60 (1.70)	0.0001
18:1ω9 (oleic)	10.8 (4.10)	12.9 (3.20)	0.0001
18:2ω6 (linoleic)	5.30 (2.80)	3.60 (1.20)	0.0001
18:3ω3 (α-linolenic)	0.29 (0.19)	0.84 (0.46)	0.0001
Alcohol	5.98 (6.90)	5.83 (5.80)	0.80
Protein, g	16.6 (3.80)	16.2 (3.10)	0.30
Fiber, g	15.5 (6.80)	18.6 (8.10)	0.004
Cholesterol, mg	312 (180)	203 (145)	0.0001

either following a Mediterranean diet or a diet low in omega–6 fatty acids but rich in omega–3 fatty acids, the best strategy to reduce the rate of complications in patients with established CHD should be to adopt an omega–3 fatty acid-rich Mediterranean diet. Two other major components of the traditional Mediterranean diet, in addition to a low omega–6/omega–3 fatty acid ratio, are low saturated fat intake and high oleic acid intake. Patients also had to meet these two major criteria of a healthy diet. Thus, to meet the criteria of a Mediterranean diet, patients had to drastically reduce the consumption of foods rich in saturated (essentially animal) fat. Among vegetable oils, only olive oil (despite its lack of ALA) and canola oil (despite its very high amounts of LA) have a fatty acid composition in line with our strategy. Thus, the patients were advised to use both oils. Because of their high content in LA, soybean, sunflower and safflower oils should not be used daily for food preparation and salad dressing. Peanut oil is too rich in saturated fatty acids and LA, and linseed (flaxseed) oil is too rich in polyunsaturated fatty acids. In theory, the best option should be to vary the use of several oils. However, when considering the difficult conditions of everyday life for many of our patients and their families, we decided to try and simplify our advice and to recommend the exclusive use of olive and canola oils.

This strategy was quite well accepted by the French patients who, at the end of the trial, were actually following a diet whose characteristics were close to that we envisaged, in theory, as the golden standard cardioprotective diet, at least in terms of lipid nutrient composition (table 1).

This exclusive use of olive and canola oils (and of canola-oil based margarine instead of butter to spread on the bread) to prepare meals and salad was

Table 2. Plasma fatty acid differences in patients following either an experimental modified diet of Crete or a prudent Western type of diet: all the differences are statistically significant (p < 0.05)

Ratios	After 2 months			After 1 year		
	Exp. (n = 236)	West (n = 247)	Diff. %	Exp. (n = 141)	West (n = 139)	Diff. %
18:1/18:2	0.809	0.658	+23	0.799	0.668	+20
18:2/18:3	42	76	−45	44	79	−44
20:4/20:5	6.8	9.1	−25	6.2	9.1	−32

Exp. = Experimental modified diet of Crete; West = Prudent Western (West) type of diet; Diff. = plasma fatty acid differences.

18:1 is oleic acid (18:1ω9), 18:2 is linoleic acid (18:2ω6), 18:3 is alpha-linolenic acid (18:3ω3), 20:4 is arachidonic acid (20:4ω6), 20:5 is eicosapentanoic acid (20:5ω3).

The three ratios are calculated by dividing the concentration of 18:1ω9 in the plasma by that of 18:2ω6, that of 18:2ω6 by that of 18:3ω3 and finally that of 20:4ω6 by that of 20:5ω3. Then, for each ratio, the difference between the 2 groups was obtained by substracting the 2 values (Experimental minus Western) divided by the value of the Western group and then multiplied by 100 to get the result in %.

a major issue in that trial as it resulted in significant differences in the fatty acid composition (tables 2, 3) of both circulating plasma lipids (essentially lipoproteins) and cell membrane phospholipids [8]. The main differences between groups in platelet phospholipid fatty acids were not seen at the level of individual fatty acids (ALA is almost undetectable in cell membranes) but for the entire family of each group. Significant differences were also seen for the ratio of omega–6 to omega–3 fatty acids [8]. When comparing the dietary fatty acids in the two groups, control patients did consume about 0.7 g of ALA per day against about 1.8 g in the experimental group, i.e. giving an LA to ALA ratio of about 10 to 1 in controls against about 4 to 1 in the experimental group. It is noteworthy that if the risk of recurrence in the experimental group was lower than in the control group, the risk in the control group was not high compared with previous studies indicating that the 10 to 1 ratio was, in theory, not so bad. Because the Mediterranean diet tested in that trial was different from the control diet in many other aspects than the LA to ALA ratio (less saturated fat, more antioxidants from various sources, more vitamins of the B group including folic acid, more vegetable proteins, and so on), the next question was to try and specify the exact role of ALA in the cardioprotection observed in the trial. Using multivariate analyses and adjustment for several confounders, we found

Table 3. Platelet phospholipid fatty acids: the lack of significant difference between groups for the individual comparison of ω3 fatty acids is partly explained by the rather small number of measurements (about n = 50 per group)

	Exp.	West	p
Saturated fatty acids			
14:0	0.28 ± 0.01	0.31 ± 0.01	<0.05
16:0	14.70 ± 0.25	14.39 ± 0.17	NS
18:0	15.81 ± 0.17	16.35 ± 0.14	0.01
Sum	30.79 ± 0.28	31.05 ± 0.21	NS
Unsaturated fatty acids			
Omega–9 family			
18:1ω9	12.56 ± 0.32	11.64 ± 0.14	0.01
20:1ω9	0.88 ± 0.04	0.74 ± 0.03	0.01
20:3ω9	0.16 ± 0.01	0.15 ± 0.01	NS
Sum	13.50 ± 0.35	12.43 ± 0.15	0.01
Omega–6 family			
18:2ω6	5.09 ± 0.16	5.46 ± 0.17	NS
20:3ω6	1.22 ± 0.03	1.31 ± 0.05	NS
20:4ω6	25.89 ± 0.33	26.45 ± 0.28	NS
22:4ω6	2.72 ± 0.09	3.02 ± 0.10	<0.05
Sum	34.93 ± 0.42	36.26 ± 0.29	0.01
Omega–3 family			
20:5ω3	0.57 ± 0.04	0.48 ± 0.04	NS
22:5ω3	2.11 ± 0.08	1.94 ± 0.06	NS
22:6ω3	2.59 ± 0.10	2.38 ± 0.10	NS
Sum	5.27 ± 0.17	4.81 ± 0.16	0.05

Exp. = Experimental modified diet of Crete; West = Prudent Western (West) type of diet; Diff. = plasma fatty acid differences.

that the plasma ALA levels measured two months after randomisation were significantly (and inversely) associated with the risk of recurrence, and in particular of fatal recurrence [18]. It could be said, however, that it is not ALA per se that was protective but the very long-chain omega–3 fatty acids derived from ALA, eicosapentanoic and docosahexanoic acids, which were also increased in the plasma of experimental patients [15]. These very long long-chain omega–3 fatty acids have indeed been demonstrated to prevent ventricular fibrillation (VF) and sudden cardiac death (SCD) in animal experiments [19–22] and in human trials [23, 24]. However, in the Lyon trial, these fatty acids were not significantly (borderline non significant with docosahexanoic acid) associated with a lower risk, which suggests that ALA was the main protective factor. Also,

Table 4. Essential fatty acid, oleic acid, folates, arginine and methionine content of various foods (per 100 g of edible portion)

	Oleate (g)	LA (g)	ALA (g)	Arginine (mg)	Methionine (mg)	Folates (μg)
Walnut	8.8	38.1	9.1	2,278	236	100
Hazelnut	45.4	7.8	0.1	2,211	221	113
Linseed	7.4	6.6	23.4	–	–	–
Peanut	23.8	15.6	0	3,085	317	173
Butternut	10.4	33.7	8.7	4,862	611	66
Almond	33.3	10.5	0.4	2,495	227	70
Pecan nut	41.2	16	0.7	1,105	186	39
Pine nut	21.5	24.9	0.8	2,251	207	58
Macadamia	41.2	1.3	0	899	92	16
Mackerel	1.2	0.1	0.5	1,427	706	1
Salmon	1.5	0.4	0.2	1,250	620	30
Beef	6.0	0.4	0.2	1,757	712	9
Pork	1.7	0.4	0	1,749	745	6

Data from the USDA Nutrient Database (Web site) and Répertoire Général des Aliments [Favier et al: Lavoisier Editors].

a specific antiarrhythmic effect of ALA itself was reported in the animal studies where it was tested [21, 22]. It does not mean, however, that the benefits of ALA are not due, at least partly, to its conversion into very long-chain omega–3 fatty acids, and further studies are required to differentiate the individual effects of each omega–3 fatty acid in the context of myocardial ischemia and ventricular arrhythmias.

Another randomised controlled trial in which the consumption of ALA was encouraged (patients of the experimental group were advised to eat more fruit, vegetables and nuts) reported a significant reduction of the risk of cardiac events in post-AMI patients [25]. In that trial, the main source of ALA was nuts (table 4). Earlier studies on Seven Day Adventists [26] and American nurses [27] suggested that eating nuts was associated with a diminished risk of CHD. Potentially protective constituents of nuts include ALA, folates, magnesium, potassium, fibre, vitamin E, arginine [28] and favourable lysine-to-arginine and methionine-to-arginine ratios [29, 30]. These ratios have been claimed to be important in the pathogenesis of CHD, the lysine-to-arginine ratio (an indirect evaluation of the consumption of animal and vegetable proteins) being potentially involved in atherogenesis [30] and the methionine-to-arginine ratio being important for endothelial function because arginine is the precursor of NO (which protects the endothelium) and methionine is the precursor of homocysteine which is toxic for the endothelium [29]. One noteworthy point is that the fatty acid composition of the lipids in walnuts (also called *English walnut* or *noix de Grenoble* or *Californian nut*) is apparently the same on both sides of the Atlantic as the concentrations of ALA, LA and oleic acid measured in our laboratory are respectively 13.4, 60.5 and 15.6% in the *noix de Grenoble* and 12.9, 62.5 and 13% in the *Californian nut*.

In table 4, the contents of the various nuts in two major amino acids, arginine (the precursor of nitric oxide) and methionine (the precursor of homocysteine), are indicated because of their importance in cardiovascular physiology and pathophysiology. They are compared with that of meat (beef and pork) and fatty fish (salmon and mackerel), which are the main sources of proteins and indispensable amino acids in the Western diet. Folic acid is also indicated because of its importance in these pathways: for the retro-conversion of homocysteine to methionine on one side, and for the recycling of tetrahydrobiopterin (which is folic acid dependent), which may account for a dysfunction of nitric oxide synthase when its availability is reduced on the other side. It is clear from table 4 that besides their fatty acid composition, certain nuts may be important because they provide large amounts of arginine (even more than meat) with the major advantage that they are quite poor in methionine (the precursor of the vasculo-toxic homocysteine) as compared with meat and fish. This is especially true for walnuts, almonds and hazelnuts, which are habitually eaten in great amounts by Mediterranean populations. The last, but certainly not least, point is the high content in folates of most nuts. Low serum folate levels [31] and high homocysteine levels [32] have been clearly associated with an increased risk of CHD. The results of recent trials, consistent with a decreased risk of CHD following homocysteine-lowering treatment with folic acid (plus vitamin B_6 or plus vitamin B_6 and vitamin B_{12}), suggest a causal relationship between low folic acid-high homocysteine and CHD [33, 34]. Thus, although there is no room here to fully discuss each of these points, nuts (which are both rich in ALA and important in the Mediterranean diet) can obviously be included as part of a healthy diet. Finally, linseed oil, with its very high content in ALA, is not advisable because of its excessive total polyunsaturated fatty acid content (LA plus ALA). As outlined [11], despite their cardioprotective properties when given in small amounts, omega–3 fatty acids, as well as polyunsaturated fatty acids in general, should not be given in large amounts: 'small is beautiful'. Thus, when considering a given food and its potentially protective constituents, we must also look at the other, potentially harmful (depending on the doses), components. Good examples are fish and fish oil. When taken in moderation, for example in DART and GISSI [23, 24], they are cardioprotective. In contrast, when taken in large doses in a low-risk population, they did not appear to be protective [35].

There are different ways to obtain 1.8–2 g of ALA per day in the diet without using ALA-containing capsules or fortified foods. The simplest (and easiest) way is to use canola oil for food preparation and salad dressing. Since 100 g of canola oil provide about 8 g of ALA, two small (US) tablespoons provide about 2 g of ALA. The canola-oil-based margarine, which contains about 5 g of ALA per 100 g of margarine, may be useful. Obtaining 2 g of ALA requires 35 g of margarine, i.e. about six teaspoons. Alternatively, one can have one tablespoon of canola oil (with salad, for instance) and 2 teaspoons of canola margarine with a piece of bread. Both canola oil and margarine can be used in association with olive oil (that does not contain ALA) for food preparation because of the large amounts of oleic acid and flavonoids it contains, and also because of its particular taste. Regarding nuts, to obtain 2 g of ALA, 4–5 English walnuts (or *noix de Grenoble*) are needed. If one likes English walnuts enough to eat them every day (as Mediterranean people used to do), it is possible to use exclusively olive oil for food preparation. A good (and definitely tasty) way is to add the nuts to salad. One can also use ground linseeds (not linseed oil) with salad or other green leafy vegetables, knowing that 100 g of ground linseeds provide about 23 g of ALA. Thus, only one tablespoon of ground linseeds provides about 2 g of ALA.

Eating purslane (or other equivalent ALA-rich leafy vegetables) to obtain large amounts of ALA is less easy, in particular because purslane (or its equivalents) is not available in many areas. In addition, one big portion (100 g of purslane) provides less than 0.4 g of ALA. Thus, for most adults, purslane should be associated with either walnuts or a salad dressing containing canola oil. One advantage of eating green leafy vegetables (and not only purslane) is to increase the diversity of the diet, which is probably a major component of any healthy diet [3]. For those who think that it is easier to take ALA supplements (capsules, for instance) rather than ALA-rich foods, it is important to remember that nutrients are not drugs. This means that when we eat foods, we eat a combination of nutrients whose proportions are not the result of chance but the product of a very long natural evolution. For instance, the proportions of certain PUFAs and many different antioxidants in a given food are probably the best combination to protect the PUFAs against peroxidation.

Fish Oil and Very Long-Chain Omega–3 Fatty Acids in Clinical Trials

The theory that eating fish may protect against SCD is derived from the results of a secondary prevention trial, the Diet And Reinfarction Trial (DART), which showed a significant reduction in total and CV mortality (both by about 30%) in patients who consumed at least 2 servings of fatty fish per week [23]. The authors suggested that the protective effect of fish might result from a preventive effect on ventricular fibrillation (VF), since no benefit was observed on the incidence of nonfatal AMI. The hypothesis was consistent with experimental evidence suggesting that the very long-chain omega–3 fatty acids, the dominant fatty acids in fish oil and fatty fish, have an important effect on the occurrence of VF in the setting of myocardial ischemia and reperfusion in various animal models, both in vivo and in vitro [19–22]. Recently, Billman et al. [22], using an elegant in vivo model of SCD in dogs, demonstrated a striking reduction of VF after intravenous administration of pure omega–3 fatty acids, including the very long-chain fatty acids present in fish oil and alpha-linolenic acid, their parent omega–3 fatty acid occurring in some vegetable oils. These authors have found the mechanism of this protection to result from the electrophysiological effects of free omega–3 fatty acids when they are simply partitioned into sarcolemma phospholipids without covalently bonding to any constituents of the cell membrane. After dietary intake, these fatty acids are preferentially incorporated into membrane phospholipids. Nair and colleagues have also shown that a considerable pool of free (non-esterified) fatty acids exists in the normal myocardium and that the amounts of omega–3 fatty acids in this pool can be increased by supplementing the diet in omega–3 fatty acids [5].

Another important aspect of the involvement of omega–3 fatty acids in SCD concerns their role in the metabolism of eicosanoids. In competition with omega–6 fatty acids, they are the precursors to a broad array of structurally diverse and potent bioactive lipids (including eicosanoids, prostaglandins and thromboxanes), which are thought to play a role in the occurrence of VF during myocardial ischemia and reperfusion [37, 38]. The exact mechanisms are not known, but an alteration of the myocardial metabolism of these compounds (for instance by aspirin blocking the first step of eicosanoid biosynthesis) may favour the occurrence of SCD in certain conditions.

Other interesting clinical data show suppression (by more than 70%) of ventricular premature complexes in middle-aged patients with frequent ventricular extrasystoles randomly assigned to take either fish oil or placebo [39]. Also, survivors of AMI [40] and healthy men [41] receiving fish oil were shown to improve their measurements of heart rate variability, which suggests that there are other mechanisms by which omega–3 fatty acids may be antiarrhythmic. In fact, parasympathetic cardiac tone is thought to provide protection against VF [42].

Support for the hypothesis of a clinically significant antiarrhythmic effect of omega–3 fatty acids in secondary prevention of CHD, as put forward in DART [23], came from the population-based case-control study conducted by Siscovick et al. [43] on the intake of omega–3 fatty acids among patients with primary cardiac arrest, in comparison with that of age- and sex-matched controls. Their data indicated that the intake of about 5–6 g of very long-chain omega–3 fatty acids per month (an amount provided by consuming fatty fish once or twice a week) was associated with a 50% reduction in the risk of cardiac arrest. In that study, the use of a biomarker – the red blood cell membrane level of omega–3 fatty acids – considerably enhanced the validity of the findings, which were also consistent with results of many (but not all) cohort studies suggesting that the consumption of one to two servings of fish per week is associated with a marked reduction in CHD mortality when compared to no fish intake [44, 45]. In most studies, however, the endpoint SCD is not reported. In a large prospective study (more than 20,000 participants with a follow-up of 11 years), Albert et al. [46] examined whether fish might have antiarrhythmic properties and prevent SCD. They found that the risk of SCD was 50% lower for men who consumed fish at least once a week than for those who had fish less than once a month. Interestingly, the consumption of fish was not related to non-sudden cardiac death, which suggests that the main protective effect of fish (or very long-chain omega–3 fatty acids) is related to an effect on arrhythmia. These results are consistent with those of DART [23] but differ from those of the Chicago Western Electric Study, in which there was a significant inverse association between fish consumption and non-sudden cardiac death, but not with SCD [47]. Several methodological factors may explain the discrepancy between the two studies, especially the way of classifying deaths in the Western Electric Study [48]. This again illustrates the limitations of observational studies and the obvious fact that only randomised trials can definitely provide a clear demonstration of causal relationships.

The GISSI-Prevenzione trial was aimed at helping in addressing the question of the health benefits of foods rich in very long-chain omega–3 fatty acids (and also in vitamin E) and their pharmacological substitutes [24]. Patients (n = 11,324) surviving a recent AMI (<3 months) were randomly assigned supplements of omega–3 fatty acids (1 g daily), vitamin E (300 mg daily), both or none (control) for 3.5 years. The primary efficacy endpoint was the combination of death and non-fatal AMI and stroke. Secondary analyses included overall mortality, CV mortality and SCD. Treatment with omega–3 fatty acids significantly lowered the risk of the primary endpoint (the relative risk decreased by 15%). Secondary analyses provided a clearer profile of the clinical effects of omega–3 fatty acids. Overall mortality was reduced by 20% and CV mortality by 30%. However, it was the effect on SCD (45% lower) that accounted for most of the benefits seen in the primary combined endpoint and both overall and CV mortality. There was no difference across the treatment

Table 5. Plasma concentrations (in % of total fatty acids) in 3 populations studied in the European IMMIDIET Project (preliminary unpublished data)

	Belgium	UK	Italy
Total fatty acids, (micro M/L)	10,342	10,579	11,111
Saturated, %	28.4	29.1	28.8
Total MUFAs, %	22.7	24.7	29.1
Total PUFAs, %	48.3	45.5	41.6
Trans fatty acids, %	0.48	0.53	0.29
Omega–3 PUFAs, %	4.8	5.4	3.8
Omega–6 PUFAs, %	43.5	40.0	37.8
Omega–6/omega–3 ratio	9.06	7.41	9.9

These data suggest that blood monounsaturated fatty acid (MUFA) levels are higher among the Italian population than among British and Belgian subjects. At the same time, Italians do have lower levels of polyunsaturated fatty acids (PUFA), trans fatty acids, ω6 and ω3 fatty acids. Thus, supplementing Italians with ω3 fatty acids is expected to result in significant benefits whereas for the British, who already have high levels in ω3 fatty acids, it is not sure whether 1g per day of very long-chain ω3 fatty acids would considerably change either blood concentrations in ω3 fatty acids or the patients' prognosis.

groups for nonfatal CV events, a result comparable to that of DART [23]. Thus, the results of that randomised trial are consistent with previous controlled trials [18, 23], large-scale observational studies [44–47] and experimental studies [19–22] which together strongly support an effect of omega–3 fatty acids in relation with SCD. A major point is that in that trial conducted in Italy, all patients were advised to follow a Mediterranean type of diet after their AMI. In their report, the GISSI investigators confirmed that the patients of both groups actually did so; for instance, more than 80% reported that they consumed olive oil every day [24]. Thus, we can say that in GISSI, the prevention of SCD resulting from the consumption of 1 g very long-chain omega–3 fatty acids was observed in patients following a Mediterranean diet as background diet. Whether they would have been protected in the same way with a non-Mediterranean diet is an open question. Another way of seeing the question is to ask whether or not the GISSI patients were relatively deficient in very long-chain omega–3 fatty acids. If they were, we can understand that even a small dose of omega–3 fatty acids was so effective. In fact, recent [unpubl.] data from the European IMMIDIET Project suggest that the Italian population could be relatively deficient in omega–3 fatty acids as compared with British (South of London) and Belgian (Flemish) populations (table 5), thus confirming the hypothesis that a low dose of omega–3 fatty acids was so effective in GISSI

Table 6. Description of the experimental and control diets in the Indo-Mediterranean Diet Heart Study

	Experimental		Control	
	baseline	2 years	baseline	2 years
Total energy, kcal	2,159	2,015	2,170	2,089
Total PUFAs, %	7.5	8.1	7.4	7.4
Total PUFAs, g	17.9	18.1	17.8	17.2
Omega–3, g	0.46	1.79	0.53	0.78
Omega–6, g	17.5	16.4	17.3	16.4
Omega–6/omega–3 ratio	38.1	9.1	32.7	21.0

because the tested population was probably relatively deficient in omega–3 fatty acids. Thus, in the context of a diet rich in oleic acid and poor in saturated and omega–6 fatty acids, even a small dose of omega–3 fatty acids (under the form of capsules) might be very protective. It is not sure whether the results would have been similar in another context, for instance in populations with high intake in omega–6 fatty acids or high intake in saturated fats.

In that regard, a recent publication [49] brings important new information about the importance of an adequate balance between omega–6 and omega–3 dietary fatty acids. Singh et al. [49] report the results of a randomised trial in secondary prevention of CHD conducted in South Asian people, a population known to be at a high risk of CHD not explained by conventional risk factors. Most randomised patients were vegetarians and did not eat fish or foods providing them with very long-chain omega–3 fatty acids. The experimental group ate more fruits, vegetables, legumes, walnuts and almonds than did controls. Also, the experimental group had an increased intake of whole grains and mustard or soybean oil that are rich in ALA. The investigators calculated that the mean intake of ALA was twice as high in the experimental group (1.8 vs. 0.8 g among controls).

The total cardiac endpoints were significantly fewer (39 vs. 76 events in controls) in the experimental group, but the difference between groups for total and cardiovascular mortality was non-significant. Thus, the intervention was less effective than in the GISSI and the Lyon trials. How can we explain such a difference when the ALA intake was comparable to that reported in the Lyon trial? A possible explanation is that the intake in omega–6 fatty acids was too high. In fact, if we calculate (table 6) the omega–6/omega–3 ratio before and after the intervention in the two groups of the Indo-Mediterranean trial [49], we observe that it was 38 and 33 before the intervention and 9 (experimental) and

21 (control) after 2 years. Thus, the ratio was still rather high in the experimental group (as high as in the control group of the Lyon trial), and this may explain why the patients did not get the maximum benefit from their experimental diet despite an increased intake in ALA. In the Lyon trial, that ratio was 4 in the experimental group and scientists recommend a ratio of 2 or even 1. The use of mustard and soybean oils in the experimental group of the Indo-Mediterranean trial probably explains that the omega–6/omega–3 ratio remained high, since soybean oil, in particular, is very rich in omega–6 fatty acids, especially LA.

A possible lesson from that trial is therefore that it is important to decrease the intake in omega–6 fatty acids when we try increasing the intake of omega–3 fatty acids to design a dietary intervention aimed at preventing fatal manifestations of CHD, as it has been done in the Lyon trial. This hypothesis remains to be confirmed. Also to be confirmed the theory that a cardioprotective diet rich in omega–3 fatty acids, can be rich in either ALA or very long-chain omega–3 fatty acids (EPA + DHA) or, alternatively, rich in either EPA or DHA. The underlying question is whether the different major omega–3 fatty acids, ALA, EPA and DHA, individually have the same cardioprotective properties. Another major unsolved question is what is the actual effectiveness of the endogenous synthesis of DHA from EPA and ALA; and whether this synthesis occurs in the same way in the different organs in humans. Recent data suggest that in humans, if any synthesis of DHA occurs from EPA or ALA, it is in small amounts [15–18, 50–52]. Our last and major question for future work is whether an increased intake of ALA and DHA (in the context of a Mediterranean diet) could be more protective than a simple increased intake in ALA, as we did in the Lyon trial [15–18].

Conclusions

The main comment in conclusion of the present review is that the intake of the different types of fatty acids is likely more a question of balance between the different families rather than a question of absolute amounts in the diet, even when these amounts are expressed in percent of total energy intake (which takes into account the level of physical exercise and the weight or body mass index of each individual). We have learnt from old studies and trials that the polyunsaturated to saturated fatty acid ratio (P/S ratio) is a very important risk factor: either too low or too high and the incidence of CHD is high [14]. From more recent studies, we are learning that the omega–6/omega–3 fatty acid ratio also is important for the prevention of CHD. The respective contribution of the different omega–3 fatty acids deserves further investigation.

References

1   Kulmacz RJ, Pendleton RB, Lands WM: Interaction between peroxidase and cyclooxygenase activities in prostaglandin-endoperoxide synthase. J Biol Chem 1994;269:5527–5536.

2   Malkowski MG, Thuresson ED, Lakkides KM, et al: Structure of eicosapentanoic and linoleic acids in the cyclooxygenase site of prostaglandin endoperoxide H synthase-1. J Biol Chem 2001; 276:37547–37555.

3   Connor WE, Neuringer M, Reisbick S: Essential fatty acids: the importance of n-3 fatty acids in the retina and brain. Nutr Rev 1992;50:21–29.

4   Neuringer M, Connor WE, Lin DS, Barstad L, Luck S: Biochemical and functional effects of prenatal and postnatal omega–3 fatty acid deficiency on retina and brain in rhesus monkeys. Proc Natl Acad Sci USA 1986;83:4021–4025.

5   Nair SD, Leitch J, Falconer J, Garg ML: Cardiac (n-3) non-esterified fatty acids are selectively increased in fish oil-fed pigs following myocardial ischemia. J Nutr 1999;129:1518–1523.

6   Connor WE. Alpha-linolenic acid in health and disease. Am J Clin Nutr 1999;69:827–828.

7   Emken EA, Adolf RO, Rakoff H, Rohwedder WK: Metabolism of deuterium-labeled linolenic, linoleic, oleic, stearic and palmitic acid in human subjects; in Baillie TA, Jones JR (eds): Synthesis and Applications of Isotopically Labeled Compounds. Amsterdam, Elsevier, 1989, pp 713–716.

8   de Lorgeril M, Salen P: Modified Mediterranean diet in the prevention of coronary heart disease and cancer. World Rev Nutr Diet. Basel, Karger, 2000, vol 87, pp 1–23.

9   Sandker GN, Kromhout D, Aravanis C, et al: Serum cholesteryl ester fatty acids and their relation with serum lipids in elderly men in Crete and Netherlands. Eur J Clin Nutr 1993;47:201–208.

10 Simopoulos AP, Norman HA, Gillapsy JE, Duke JA: Common purslane: a source of omega–3 fatty acids and antioxidants. J Am Coll Nutr 1992;11:374–382.

11 Simopoulos AP, Salem N: n-3 fatty acids in eggs from range-fed Greek chickens. N Engl J Med 1989;321:1412.

12 Renaud S: Linoleic acid, platelet aggregation and myocardial infarction. Atherosclerosis 1990;80: 255–256.

13 Renaud S, Nordoy A: Small is beautiful: Alpha-linolenic and eicosapentanoic acids in man. Lancet 1983;i:1169.

14 Renaud S, de Lorgeril M: Dietary lipids and their relation to ischemic heart disease: From epidemiology to prevention. J Intern Med 1989;225:39–46.

15 de Lorgeril M, Renaud S, Mamelle N, et al: Mediterranean alpha-linolenic acid-rich diet in secondary prevention of coronary heart disease. Lancet 1994;343:1454–1459.

16 de Lorgeril M, Salen P, Martin JL, et al: Effect of a Mediterranean-type of diet on the rate of cardiovascular complications in coronary patients: Insights into the cardioprotective effect of certain nutriments. J Am Coll Cardiol 1996;28:1103–1108.

17 de Lorgeril M, Salen P, Caillat-Vallet E, et al: Control of bias in dietary trial to prevent coronary recurrences. The Lyon Diet Heart Study. Eur J Clin Nutr 1997;51:116–122.

18 de Lorgeril M, Salen P, Martin JL, et al: Mediterranean diet, traditional risk factors and the rate of cardiovascular complications after myocardial infarction. Final report of the Lyon Diet Heart Study. Circulation 1999;99:779–785.

19 McLennan PL, Abeywardena MY, Charnock JS: Reversal of arrhythmogenic effects of long term saturated fatty acid intake by dietary n-3 and n-6 polyunsaturated fatty acids. Am J Clin Nutr 1990;51:53–58.

20 McLennan PL, Abeywardena MY, Charnock JS: Dietary fish oil prevents ventricular fibrillation following coronary occlusion and reperfusion. Am Heart J 1988;16:709–716.

21 Isensee H, Jacob R: Differential effects of various oil diets on the risk of cardiac arrhythmias in rats. J Cardiovasc Risk 1994;1:353–359.

22 Billman GE, Kang JX, Leaf A: Prevention of sudden cardiac death by dietary pure omega–3 polyunsaturated fatty acids in dogs. Circulation 1999;99:2452–2457.

23 Burr ML, Fehily AM, Gilbert JF, et al: Effects of changes in fat, fish, and fibre intakes on death and myocardial reinfarction: Diet and Reinfarction Trial (DART). Lancet 1989;ii:757–761.

24 GISSI-Prevenzione Investigators: Dietary supplementation with n-3 polyunsaturated fatty acids and vitamin E after myocardial infarction: Results of the GISSI-Prevenzione trial. Lancet 1999; 354:447–455.

25 Singh RB, Rastogi SS, Verma R, Laxmi B, Singh R, Ghosh S, Niaz MA: Randomised controlled trial of cardioprotective diet in patients with recent acute myocardial infarction: Results of one year follow-up. BMJ 1992;304:1015–1019.

26 Fraser GE, Sabaté J, Beeson WL, Strahan TM: A possible protective effect of nut consumption on risk of coronary heart disease. Arch Intern Med 1992;152:1416–1424.

27 Hu FB, Stampfer MJ, Manson JE, et al: Frequent nut consumption and risk of coronary heart disease in women: prospective cohort study. BMJ 1998;317:1341–1345.

28 Cooke JP, Tsao P, Singer A, et al: Anti-atherogenic effect of nuts: is the answer NO? Arch Intern Med 1993;153:896–897.

29 de Lorgeril M: Dietary arginine in prevention of cardiovascular diseases. Cardiovasc Res 1998;37: 560–563.

30 Kritchevski D, Tepper SA, Czarnecki SK, Klurfeld DM: Atherogenicity of animal and vegetable protein: influence of the lysine to arginine ratio. Atherosclerosis 1982;41:429–431.

31 Robinson K, Arheart K, Refsum H, et al: Low circulating folate and vitamin B_6 concentrations: Risk factors for stroke, peripheral vascular disease and coronary heart disease. Circulation 1998; 97:437–443.

32 Bostom AG, Selhub J: Homocysteine and arteriosclerosis. Subclinical and clinical disease associations. Circulation 1999;99:2361–2363.

33 Vermeulen EG, Stehouwer CD, Twisk JW, et al: Effect of homocysteine-lowering treatment with folic acid plus vitamin B_6 on progression of subclinical atherosclerosis: a randomised, placebo-controlled trial. Lancet 2000;355:517–522.

34 Schnyder G, Roffi M, Flammer Y, et al: Effect of homocysteine-lowering therapy with folic acid, vitamin B_{12}, and vitamin B_6 on clinical outcome after percutaneous coronary intervention. The Swiss Heart Study: A randomised controlled trial. JAMA 2002;288:973–979.

35 Marckmann P, Gronbaek M: Fish consumption and coronary heart disease mortality. A systematic review of prospective cohort studies. Eur J Clin Nutr 1999;53:585–590.

36 Kant AK, Schatzkin A, Ziegler RG: Dietary diversity and subsequent cause-specific mortality in the NHANES I Epidemiologic Follow-up Study. J Am Coll Nutr 1995;14:233–238.

37 Corr PB, Saffitz JE, Sobel BE: What is the contribution of altered lipid metabolism to arrhythmogenesis in the ischemic heart? in Hearse DJ, Manning AS, Janse MJ (eds): Life Threatening Arrhythmias during Ischemia and Infarction. New York, Raven Press, 1987, pp 91–114.

38 Parratt JR, Coker SJ, Wainwright CL: Eicosanoids and susceptibility to ventricular arrhythmias during myocardial ischemia and reperfusion. J Mol Cell Cardiol 1987;19(suppl 5):55–66.

39 Sellmayer A, Witzgall H, Lorenz RL, et al: Effects of dietary fish oil on ventricular premature complexes. Am J Cardiol 1995;76:974–977.

40 Christensen JH, Gustenhoff P, Korup E, et al: Effect of fish oil on heart rate variability in survivors of myocardial infarction: A double blind randomised controlled trial. BMJ 1996;312:677–678.

41 Christensen JH, Christensen MS, Dyerberg J, et al: Heart rate variability and fatty acid content of blood cell membranes: a dose-response study with n-3 fatty acids. Am J Clin Nutr 1999;70: 331–337.

42 Farrell TG, Bashir Y, Cripps T, et al: Risk stratification for arrhythmic events in postinfarction patients based on heart rate variability, ambulatory electrocardiographic variables and the signal-averaged electrocardiogram. J Am Coll Cardiol 1991;18:687–697.

43 Siscovick DS, Raghunathan TE, King I, et al: Dietary intake and cell membrane levels of long-chain n-3 polyunsaturated fatty acids and the risk of primary cardiac arrest. JAMA 1995;274: 1363–1367.

44 Kromhout D, Bosschieter EB, de Lezenne Coulander C: The inverse relation between fish consumption and 20-year mortality from coronary heart disease. N Engl J Med 1985;312:1205–1209.

45 Shekelle RB, Missel L, Paul O, et al: Fish consumption and mortality from coronary heart disease. N Engl J Med 1985;313:820.

46 Albert CM, Hennekens CH, O'Donnel CJ, et al: Fish consumption and the risk of sudden cardiac death. JAMA 1998;279:23–28.

47   Daviglus ML, Stamler J, Orencia AJ, et al: Fish consumption and the 30-year risk of fatal myo-
     cardial infarction. N Engl J Med 1997;336:1046–1053.
48   Albert CA, Manson JE, Hennekens CH: Fish consumption and the risk of myocardial infarction.
     N Engl J Med 1997;337:497.
49   Singh RB, Dubnov G, Niaz M, et al: Effect of an Indo-Mediterranean diet on progression of coro-
     nary artery disease in high-risk patients (Indo-Mediterranean Diet Heart Study): A randomised
     single-blind trial. Lancet 2002;360:1455–1461.
50   Li D, Sinclair A, Wilson A, et al: Effect of dietary alpha-linolenic acid on thrombotic risk factors
     in vegetarian men. Am J Clin Nutr 1999;69:872–882.
51   Mantzioris E, James MJ, Gibson RA, Cleland LG: Dietary substitution with an alpha-linolenic
     acid-rich vegetable oil increases eicosapentanoic acid concentrations in tissues. Am J Clin Nutr
     1994;59:1304–1309.
52   Kwon JS, Snook JT, Wardlaw GM, Hwang DH: Effects of diets high in saturated fatty acids,
     canola oil, or safflower oil on platelet function, thromboxane B_2 formation, and fatty acid
     composition of platelet phospholipids. Am J Clin Nutr 1991;54:351–358.

Dr. M. de Lorgeril
Laboratoire du Stress Cardiovasculaire et Pathologies Associées
UFR de Médecine et Pharmacie, Domaine de la Merci
F–38706 La Tronche (Grenoble) (France)
E-Mail michel.delorgeril@ujf-grenoble.fr

Simopoulos AP, Cleland LG (eds): Omega–6/Omega–3 Essential Fatty Acid Ratio:
The Scientific Evidence. World Rev Nutr Diet. Basel, Karger, 2003, vol 92, pp 74–80

....

Effects of an Indo-Mediterranean Diet on the Omega–6/Omega–3 Ratio in Patients at High Risk of Coronary Artery Disease: The Indian Paradox

Daniel Pella[a], Gal Dubnov[b], Ram B. Singh[c], Rakesh Sharma[d],
Elliot M. Berry[b], Orly Manor[b]

[a] 2nd Interna Klinika,Safaric University, Kosice, Slovakia;
[b] Department of Human Nutrition and Metabolism, Hebrew University, Hadassah
Medical School, Jerusalem, Israel;
[c] Subharti Medical College, Medical Hospital and Research Centre, Moradabad, India;
[d] Department of Medicine, Columbia University, New York, N.Y., USA

Coronary artery disease (CAD) has become a major health problem in the Western world, and is rapidly increasing in the developing countries, accompanied by rapid changes in diet and lifestyle [1–3]. The prevalence of CAD is 2–3% in rural areas and 9–14% in urban populations of India [2, 3]. This finding is associated with a lower total fat intake in rural areas compared to urban ones (10–15 vs. 15–27 en %/day, respectively) [2–4]. The paradox is that despite low fat intake relative to Western countries, the urban population has a high prevalence of CAD. The rural population in north and east India consumes more mustard oil and grains, which are considered a poor man's food. In urban areas, Indian ghee (clarified butter rich in cholesterol oxide [5]), vegetable ghee, butter, cream, refined oils and refined bread and flour are substituted for mustard oils and whole grains, resulting in marked changes in the omega–6/ omega–3 ratio of urban diets [2–4]. The cause of the Indian paradox can be explained by the increased ratio of omega–6/omega–3 fatty acids in the urban diets.

The dietary changes described are more pronounced in patients with high risk of CAD [4, 6–11]. It is possible that decreased consumption of omega–3 fatty acids may increase the coronary risk among urban subjects and in patients with CAD. Supplementation with foods rich in alpha-linolenic acid, a plant-derived omega–3 fatty acid, such as mustard oil, soy bean oil, whole grains, walnuts, fruits and vegetables, may enhance alpha-linolenic acid content in the diet. This will decrease the dietary omega–6/omega–3 ratio, now believed to be protective against CAD [6–10].

Fat Intake and Disease in Rural, Urban and Immigrant Indians

Among immigrant Indians to the western world, and among Indians living in the urban setting, CAD prevalence and mortality are higher than expected [4, 12]. This increased morbidity is not explained by the conventional risk factors alone [2, 13, 14], and the importance of dietary fat intake has emerged as a possible explanation. Additional findings, such as elevated CRP and homocysteine levels among Indian immigrants to the UK [15, 16] may suggest other dietary factors as possible targets for nutritional modification.

In a population survey of 162 rural and 152 urban subjects aged 26–65 years in north India, the findings are compared with existing data on Indian immigrants to the United Kingdom and the United States [4]. In comparison with rural subjects, the urban population had a higher prevalence of CAD (8.6 vs. 3.0%) and type 2 diabetes (7.9 vs. 2.5%), higher blood pressure, total and low density lipoprotein cholesterol, triglycerides and postprandial 2-hour blood glucose and plasma insulin. These observations are similar to the observations made in UK among Indians compared to Caucasians living in London [4]. The urban subjects were eating higher total and saturated fat, cholesterol and refined carbohydrates and lower total and complex carbohydrates compared to rurals of both genders. Omega–6/omega–3 fatty acid ratio was significantly lower in the rural population compared to the urban one (table 1). In Indian immigrants to the UK and the USA, the omega–6/omega–3 ratios were 16:1 and 15:1; values are higher than those in British natives (6:1) [17]. In subjects with CAD risk factors, omega–6/omega–3 fat ratios were also higher, when compared to those in subjects without these risk factors, as shown in table 2 [4].

The Indian Lifestyle and Heart Study in Elderly, conducted among 515 rural and 595 urban Indian subjects aged 50 years and above, showed interesting findings related to fatty acid consumption [11]. The omega–6/omega–3 fat ratio among rural elderly subjects was only 4.4:1 (table 3). The total prevalence of CAD, based on a clinical history and an electrocardiogram, was significantly higher among the urban population than it was among rural subjects aged 50–84 years (12.1 vs. 4.0%). The rates were comparable in the two genders, but increased with age. In comparison with rural subjects, the urban subjects had a 2- to 3-fold higher prevalence of hypertension, type 2 diabetes, hypercholesterolemia, hypertriglyceridemia, overweight and central obesity. Risk factor

Table 1. Omega–6/omega–3 fat ratio in rural and urban population in relation to Indian immigrants [data from ref. 4]

Nutrient	Indian rural	Indian urban	Indian in UK	Indian in USA
n	162	152	184	1,325
Total energy, kcal/day	2,180 (170)	2,112 (162)	2,415	2,400
Total carbohydrates, en %/day	73.0 (2.5)*	62.1 (2.1)	48.6	55.0
Total protein, en %/day	12.2 (1.2)	13.2 (1.2)	12.6	13.5
Total fat, en %/day	14.8 (1.4)*	24.7 (1.5)	38.8	31.5
Saturated fat, en %/day	4.9 (0.5)*	9.2 (0.7)	13.7	10.6
Omega–6/omega–3 fat ratio	2.3 (0.3)*	6.2 (0.6)	16.0	15.0
Total fruit, vegetable, legume, g/day	78.6 (6.5)*	120.0 (10.6)	150	150

Values are mean (SD) and p values were obtained by comparison of rural and urban subjects by analysis of variance. *$p < 0.01$.

Table 2. Omega–6/omega–3 fat ratio in the diets of subjects with coronary risk factors [data from ref. 4]

Nutrient	Diabetes[+]	Hypertension	Hypercholesterolemia	CAD	No risk
Total energy, kcal/day	2,170 (176)	2,115 (165)	2,125 (160)	2,080 (165)	2,075 (170)
Total fat, en %/day	27.8 (1.8)*	29.0 (1.8)*	28.4 (1.9)*	26.8 (1.5)*	20.5 (1.7)
Carbohydrates, en %/day	56.8 (2.2)*	56.5 (2.1)*	57.8 (2.3)*	58.2 (2.4)*	66.2 (2.8)
Saturated fat, en %/day	10.5 (1.2)*	10.7 (1.2)*	10.9 (1.4)*	9.8 (1.2)*	6.8 (1.0)
Omega–6/ omega–3 ratio	5.6 (1.8)*	6.8 (2.1)*	6.9 (2.2)*	6.6 (2.3)*	5.6 (1.8)

Values are mean (standard deviation). p values were obtained by comparison of risk factor with no risk factor by Analysis of variance. *$p < 0.01$. [+]Includes diabetes and glucose intolerance.

levels were also significantly greater among the urban subjects than the rurals. The findings indicate that rural and urban subjects are characterized by different dietary patterns and a different omega–6/omega–3 fatty acid ratio, which may be responsible for differences in the prevalence of risk factors among these populations groups.

Table 3. Omega–6/omega–3 fat ratio in the diets of rural and urban elderly subjects [data from ref. 11]

Nutrient	Men		Women	
	rural (n = 280)	urban (n = 314)	rural (n = 235)	urban (n = 281)
Total energy, kcal/day	2,258 (161)	2,282 (180)	2,180 (160)	2,195 (164)
Total carbohydrates, en %/day	68.8 (3.8)*	59.6 (3.1)	77.8 (3.8)*	59.0 (2.8)
Total fat, en %/day	16.6 (1.8)*	26.8 (2.6)	14.6 (1.6)*	26.8 (2.8)
Saturated fat, en %/day	5.5 (1.1)*	10.8 (1.9)	5.6 (1.8)*	10.8 (1.8)
Omega–6/omega–3 fat ratio	4.4 (0.7)*	8.8 (1.7)	4.8 (0.8)*	8.4 (1.8)
Total fruit, vegetables and legumes, g/day	136.5 (14.6)*	194.8 (18.6)	118.8 (9.8)*	185.0 (16.2)

Values are mean (SD). p values were obtained by comparison of data of rural with urban subjects by analysis of variance. *$p < 0.01$.

Clinical Trials

Several clinical trials conducted among the Indian population as well as others have proven the benefit of omega–3 fatty acids. For example, the Indo-Mediterranean Diet Heart Study was a randomized, single blind trial conducted among 1,000 Indian patients with either established CAD (angina pectoris or previous myocardial infarction) or only CAD risk factors, which examined the effect of a diet rich in alpha-linolenic acid on CAD events [9]. 499 patients were administered a diet rich in whole grains, fruits, vegetables, walnuts, mustard or soy bean oil as a source for omega–3 fat; 501 subjects were advised to consume the National Cholesterol Education Program (NCEP) Step I diet prudent diet. At the end of a 2-year follow-up, the intervention group consumed significantly more fruits, vegetables and legumes than did the control group (573 ± 127 vs. 231 ± 19 g/day, $p < 0.001$), as well as more mustard and soy bean oil (31 ± 6.5 vs. 15.2 ± 5.5 g/day, $p < 0.001$). The mean intake of alpha-linolenic acid was over 2-fold greater in the intervention group compared to the control group (1.8 ± 0.4 vs. 0.8 ± 0.2 g/day, $p < 0.001$). The omega–6/omega–3 fatty acids ratio was slightly higher at baseline in the intervention group than in control group (39 ± 12 vs. 34 ± 10), yet both these figures are extremely high, reflecting a diet with a very high omega–6 content yet low omega–3. At the end of a 2-year follow-up, this ratio showed a marked decline in the intervention group, which was greater than that observed in the control group consuming the NCEP diet (9.1 ± 12 vs. 21 ± 10, $p < 0.001$). Regarding the study endpoints, total

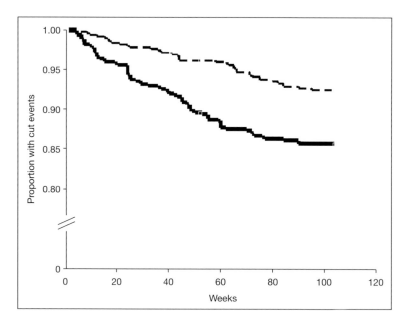

Fig. 1. Kaplan-Meier Cumulative survival curves of proportion of subjects without fatal MI, nonfatal MI, or sudden cardiac death among experimental (broken line) and control (continuous line) groups in the Indo-Mediterranean Diet Heart study. Data from Singh [9].

cardiac events were significantly fewer in the intervention group than in the controls (39 vs. 76 events, p < 0.001), as shown in figure 1. Sudden cardiac deaths were also reduced (6 vs. 16, p = 0.015), as were nonfatal myocardial infarctions (21 vs. 43, p < 0.001). These findings show that dietary changes may induce a marked change in the omega–6/omega–3 fatty acid ratio. This may be associated with the large risk reduction observed. Further analysis of the fatty acid ratio and its influence on the endpoints is in progress. Still, it is apparent that the fatty acid ratio remains much higher than recommended. A value of 1–2:1 has been shown by Simopoulos [18] to be the ratio in the traditional diet of Crete, where the concept of the Mediterranean diet originated from. Recommendations from the Joint WHO/FAO Expert Consultation on Diet, Nutrition and the Prevention of Chronic Diseases suggests consuming omega–6 PUFA at 5–8% of energy and omega–3 PUFA at 1–2% of energy [19]. This results in a 'recommended' omega–6/omega–3 ratio, ranging from 2.5:1 to 8:1. Perhaps among a population with such a high dietary ratio as in the urban Indians, only a lowering of the ratio can be a goal, without aspiring to reach levels of the western world or the traditional Mediterranean area.

In another primary prevention trial carried out in the Netherlands [20], conducted among 282 subjects with multiple risk factors of CAD, Bemelmans et al. [20] evaluated the protective effects of alpha-linolenic acid on CAD and its risk factors. Alpha-linolenic acid was compared with linoleic acid (the major omega–6 fatty acid in the diet), and both fatty acids were included in the diet through special margarines. In the alpha-linolenic acid group, the intake of omega–3 fatty acids was 6.3 g/day, and that of omega–6 was 26.3 g/day; in the linoleic acid group, the intake of omega–3 fatty acids was 1 g/day, and that of omega–6 was 28.8 g/day. Plasma fibrinogen levels were lower in the omega–3 fatty acid group than in the omega–6 fatty acid group. Cardiac events were insignificantly lower in the omega–3 group than in the omega–6 group, respectively (2 vs. 9, $p < 0.20$), suggesting that a positive effect may be seen with a longer follow-up.

Conclusions

The Indian population suffers from an increased incidence of CAD despite a low-fat diet. This may be due to a diet with a very high omega–6/omega–3 ratio. The findings from the Indo-Mediterranean Diet Heart Study, as well as other intervention trials and epidemiological studies indicate that a dietary modification may induce positive changes in the dietary omega–6/omega–3 fat ratio. This is expected to translate into CAD reduction.

References

1   Nishtar S: Prevention of coronary heart disease in south Asia. Lancet 2002;360:1015–1018.
2   Singh RB, Tomlinson B, Thomas GN, Sharma RK: Coronary artery disease and coronary risk factors: The South Asian Paradox. J Nutr Environ Med 2001;11:43–51.
3   Pella D, Thomas N, Tomlinson N, Singh RB: Prevention of coronary artery disease: The South Asian paradox. Lancet 2003;361:79.
4   Singh RB, Ghosh S, Niaz AM, Gupta S, Bishnoi I, Sharma JP, Agarwal P, Rastogi SS, Beegum R, Chibo H: Epidemiologic study of diet and coronary risk factors in relation to central obesity and insulin levels in rural and urban populations of north India. Int J Cardiol 1995;47:245–255.
5   Jacobson MS: Cholesterol oxides in Indian ghee: Possible cause of unexplained high risk of atherosclerosis in Indian immigrant populations. Lancet 1987;ii:656–658.
6   Lanzaman-Petithory D, Pueyo S, Renaud S: Primary prevention of cardiovascular diseases by alpha-linolenic acid. Am J Clin Nutr 2003;76:1456–1457.
7   Renaud SC, Lanzmann-Petithory D: The beneficial effects of alpha linolenic acid in coronary artery disease is not questionable. Am J Clin Nutr 2003;76:903–904.
8   Singh RB, Niaz MA, Kartik C: Can omega–3 fatty acids provide myocardial protection by decreasing infarct size and inhibiting atherothrombosis? Eur Heart J 2001;3(suppl):62–69.
9   Singh RB, Dubnov G, Niaz MA, Saraswati Ghosh, Singh R, Rastogi SS, Manor O, Pella D, Berry EM: Effect of an Indo-Mediterranean diet on progression of coronary artery disease in high risk patients (Indo-Mediterranean Diet Heart Study): A randomised single-blind trial. Lancet 2002;360:1455–1461.

10   Thies F, Garry JM, Yaqoob P, Rerkasem K, Williams J, Shearman CP, Gallagher PJ, Calder PC, Grimble RF: Association of omega–3 fatty acids with stability of atherosclerotic plaques: A randomized controlled trial. Lancet 2003;361:477–485.

11   Singh RB, Niaz MA, Rastogi V: Prevalence of coronary artery disease and coronary risk factors in the elderly rural and urban populations of north India: The Indian Lifestyle and Heart Study in Elderly. Cardiol Elderly 1996;4:111–117.

12   Balarajan R: Ethnic differences in mortality from ischaemic heart disease and cerebrovascular disease in England and Wales. BMJ 1991;302:560–564.

13   Janus ED, Postiglione A, Singh RB, Lewis B: The modernisation of Asia. Implications for coronary heart disease. Council on Arteriosclerosis of the International Society and Federation of Cardiology. Circulation 1996;94:2671–2673.

14   McKeigue PM, Shah B, Marmot MG: Relation of central obesity and insulin resistance with high diabetes prevalence and cardiovascular risk in South Asians. Lancet 1991;337:382–386.

15   Chambers JC, Obeid OA, Refsum H, Ueland P, Hackett D, Hooper J, Turner RM, Thompson SG, Kooner JS: Plasma homocysteine concentrations and risk of coronary heart disease in UK Indian Asian and European men. Lancet 2000;355:523–527.

16   Chambers JC, Eda S, Bassett P, Karim Y, Thompson SG, Gallimore JR, Pepys MB, Kooner JS: C-reactive protein, insulin resistance, central obesity, and coronary heart disease risk in Indian Asians from the United Kingdom compared with European whites. Circulation 2001;104:145–150.

17   Singh RB, Ahmad S, Niaz MA: Research in nutrition (letter). Natl Med J India 1994;7:50.

18   Simopoulos AP: Essential fatty acids in health and chronic disease. Am J Clin Nutr 1999;70(suppl): 560s–569s.

19   World Health Organization: Diet, nutrition, and the prevention of chronic diseases.

20   Bemelmans WJ, Broer J, Feskens EJ, Smit AJ, Muskiet FA, Lefrandt JD, Bom VJ, May JF, Meyboom-de Jong B: Effect of an increased intake of alpha-linolenic acid and group nutritional education on the cardiovascular risk factors: The Mediterranean Alpha-Linolenic Enriched Groningen Dietary Intervention (MARGARIN) Study. Am J Clin Nutr 2002;75:221–227.

Dr. R.B. Singh, MD, Subharti Medical College
Medical Hospital and Research Centre
Civil Lines, Moradabad-10(UP)244001 (India)
E-Mail icn@mickyonline.com

Simopoulos AP, Cleland LG (eds): Omega–6/Omega–3 Essential Fatty Acid Ratio:
The Scientific Evidence. World Rev Nutr Diet. Basel, Karger, 2003, vol 92, pp 81–91

....

Omega–6/Omega–3 Fatty Acid Ratio: The Israeli Paradox

Gal Dubnov, Elliot M. Berry

Department of Human Nutrition and Metabolism, Hebrew University,
Hadassah Medical School, Jerusalem, Israel

While the *amount* of fat is very important in terms of public health in
dealing with the current epidemic of obesity, an equally significant issue is the
type of fat consumed. As polyunsaturated fatty acids (PUFA) have long been
shown to possess cholesterol-lowering effects [1], increasing their consumption
has been promoted in the management of coronary artery disease (CAD) [2].
These recommendations followed both experimental and population based
studies that showed decreasing rates of CAD in countries with increasing
polyunsaturated/saturated fat (P/S) ratios over the past years.

The dietary habits in Israel appear to be as recommended: low in total
calories, in total fat and in saturated fat, while high in hypolipidemic omega–6
fatty acids (ω6) as compared with other western countries [3, 4]. Unexpectedly, the
rates of modern-world illnesses are about the same as they are in the USA and
Europe [3, 5, 6]. The reason for this is not clear. Recent evidence suggests that
a high intake of omega–6 fatty acids may prove harmful [2, 7–9]: these fatty
acids may elevate the risk of hyperinsulinemia and its associated metabolic disorders, atherogenesis, and cancer. Another group of PUFA, the omega–3 fatty
acids (ω3), have demonstrated cardioprotection in observational [10–15] and
intervention studies for both secondary [16–18] and primary [18] prevention.
An example for this is shown in figure 1: an Indo-Mediterranean diet, rich in
the plant-derived omega–3 fatty acid alpha-linolenic acid, markedly decreased
the risk for a cardiac event among both those with established coronary artery
disease, or those only with risk factors [18]. A recent meta-analysis showed that
both dietary and non-dietary sources are equally beneficial [19], and the health
benefits of plant- derived or fish- derived omega–3 fatty acids now seem to
have a sound basis [20]. As the omega–6 and omega–3 fatty acids compete for

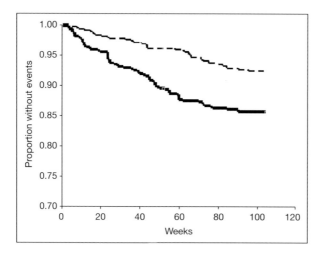

Fig. 1. Kaplan Meier cumulative survival curves of proportion of subjects without fatal MI, nonfatal MI, or sudden cardiac death among experimental (broken line) and control (continuous line) groups in the Indo-Mediterranean Diet Heart Study. The experimental group received a diet enriched with alpha-linolenic acid, a plant-derived ω–3 fatty acid. The control group was advised to consume the National Cholesterol Education Program Step I diet. The risk for cardiac events at the end of a 2-year follow-up was 50% lower in the ω–3 supplemented group. Data from Singh et al. [18].

the same enzymes in their metabolic pathways, the levels of one may influence the other. The end product of the omega–6 pathway is arachidonic acid (AA), a factor in insulin resistance and a common precursor for several pro-inflammatory and tumor- enhancing eicosanoids. The competition of omega–3 on the metabolic enzymes may therefore reduce AA levels, resulting in a lower incidence of diabetes mellitus, atherosclerosis, and cancer. This is the basis for discussion regarding the dietetic, and hence in vivo ratios between omega–6 and omega–3 fatty acids. The unexpectedly high incidence of chronic western diseases in Israel, despite a seemingly protective diet, provides evidence for the importance of the ratio or, better, the balance, between these fatty acids.

Omega–6/Omega–3 Fatty Acid Ratio

The Dangers of a High Omega–6 Intake
While considering the potential harm of omega–6 PUFA, especially the more common linoleic acid (LA, C18:2ω6), one must keep in mind that these are *essential* fatty acids, which must be consumed to ensure normal

functioning of membranes, inflammatory, immune and coagulation responses. Therefore, a range of recommended intake is usually suggested, and not only an upper limit as is given for saturated fatty acids (SFA). The recommended range of LA intake is 2–3% of total energy [21]. Though essential, there are possible dangers of high PUFA intake [2, 7–9]. Low-density lipoprotein (LDL) particles rich in omega–6 are more prone to oxidation [22]. This process may be blocked by the antioxidative properties of vitamin E, but large amounts of LA will overwhelm its protective capabilities. With the current concept that oxidized LDL is atherogenic, this process is undesirable, as it may promote atherosclerosis and CAD. Omega–6 fatty acids may also increase the secretion of insulin leading to hyperinsulinemia and insulin resistance [7]. Insulin, in turn, activates phospholipase A_2, which releases more PUFA from cell membranes. These free fatty acids act as substrates for eicosanoid formation, and some of these leukotrienes and prostaglandins are proinflammatory, thrombogenic, vasoactive, arrhythmogenic and carcinogenic. In this way, high omega–6 levels might augment the occurrence of CAD and its thrombotic events, insulin resistance and related diabetes, dyslipidemia and hypertension, and cancer. Despite these apparent detrimental effects, the original idea of the benefits of LA intake still survives: recent studies have shown that increasing LA intake was protective of CAD [23] while increased plasma levels were protective of stroke [24]. An explanation might be that the polyunsaturated fatty acids should also be considered in relation to the antioxidative (redox) status, that is in relation to vitamins E and C levels. If the latter are sufficient, then probably these beneficial effects might be dominant [25]. It should be disclosed that there are actually no convincing human studies that consumption of omega–6 fatty acids are indeed harmful.

The Omega–6/Omega–3 Ratio

It has been known for about 40 years, that alpha-linolenic acid (ALA, C18:3ω3) – the basic ω–3 fatty acid – inhibits LA metabolism into arachidonic acid (AA, C20:4ω6) [26]. Equally, LA can interfere with the metabolism of ALA, as they compete for the same enzymes. One of the first studies to discuss different ratios between these two essential fatty acids was probably that of Mohrhauer and Holman [27]. It was later determined that the omega–6/omega–3 ratio has implications in several major health conditions. Mathematically, a ratio can be enlarged either by increasing the nominator or by decreasing the denominator. Biologically, these effects are neither necessarily comparable nor equal and, because of this, some researchers do not like the term 'ratio'. However, many studies discuss the concept and therefore, in this review, it has been retained – but one should keep in mind these caveats. Given the growing evidence that omega–3 fatty acids have many health benefits [10–20, 28], it seems that decreasing the omega–6/omega–3 ratio without deliberately increasing omega–3 levels is unacceptable.

General recommendations from an international workshop devoted to this issue are to reduce plant oil-derived LA consumption, and to increase omega–3 consumption [21], attempting to reduce the omega–6/omega–3 ratio by changing both constituents of the 'ratio'. The desirable increase in omega–3 consumption is also reflected in the latest American Heart Association dietary recommendations, where at least 2 weekly servings of fish are advocated [29]. One major health problem in which this ratio is of consequence is coronary artery disease (CAD). In a prospective study that included data on LA, ALA and CAD, a modest reduction in fatal disease was shown when the LA:ALA ratio was lower than 10 [15]. It is noteworthy that this effect was less than that of the individual fatty acids alone. Data from the NHLBI Family Heart Study showed that increasing quintiles of ALA intake were protective of CAD only when the LA:ALA ratio was lower than 8.5 [23]. Here, increasing the intake of both fatty acids was beneficial; the protective effect of LA was seen even after adjustment for ALA intake.

An additional health benefit of a decreased omega–6/omega–3 ratio is a reduction in carcinogenesis [9]. The suggested mechanism involves the attenuation of AA production, and hence its carcinogenic metabolites. This is the case, for example, of breast cancer [30]. A study of breast adipose tissue from either breast cancer patients or those with benign disease showed a 60% lower adjusted risk of cancer in patients in the lowest vs. highest tertiles of omega–6/omega–3 ratios [31]. While tertile cutoff points were not given, the average omega–6/omega–3 ratio in cases and controls was around 15–16:1. A ratio of 1–2:1 is suggested as that which best suppresses growth and development of this tumor [32].

Another emerging health benefit of a low omega–6/omega–3 ratio lies in bone turnover: animal studies show that a low omega–6/omega–3 ratio has beneficial effects on bone mineral density [33]. Only 3 human studies conducted so far had contradictory results [34–36], so a final verdict in this matter is not yet available.

The optimal omega–6/omega–3 ratio is not known. A value of 1–2:1 has been shown by Simopoulos [37] to be the ratio in the traditional diet of Crete, which is consistent with the estimates of the Paleolithic diet by Eaton et al. [38], yet this could be an unachievable goal in modern western nutrition. National and international recommendations range from 2:1 in Japan and 2.3:1 in USA, to 5:1 in Sweden and, until recently, 5–10:1 by the WHO [39]. Current recommendations from the Joint WHO/FAO Expert Consultation on Diet, Nutrition and the Prevention of Chronic Diseases suggests consuming omega–6 PUFA at 5–8% of energy, omega–3 PUFA at 1–2% of energy – hence ratios would be expected to range 2.5:1 to 8:1 [40]. The way of reaching these values would be a reduction in LA (only in those areas with excess intake) and increasing nut, oil, and fish intake as sources of omega–3 [21]. It is noteworthy that essentially all foods containing LA, ALA (or both), affect the dietary omega–6/omega–3 ratio, and not only from oils. Walnuts, a food component repeatedly shown to have cardioprotective properties, have an LA:ALA ratio of 4.2 [41]. This is due to the much higher content of ALA (9 g/100 g edible portion) as compared with other common types of nuts. Therefore, even a hypothetical diet of walnuts alone would not bring this ratio to its minimum. The meat of beef fed on grass had an omega–6/omega–3 ratio of 2:1, while that of grain-fed beef, as modern cattle is raised, has a ratio of 15:1 [9]. This same concept occurs in humans as 'we are what we eat'. Another interesting fact is the LA:ALA ratio in, for example, eggs: while US eggs have about 60% more LA, Greek eggs have 1.300% more ALA, resulting in a much more favorable LA:ALA ratio (2.3:1 in Greece, but 50:1 in USA supermarkets) [32]. The total omega–6/omega–3 ratio in these eggs is 1.3:1 in Greece, but 19.4:1 in the USA. In sum, altering the balance between these fatty acids in a population might require changes in many nutrient sources; it seems that the diet recommended by many organizations to be rich in fruit, vegetables, whole grains, nuts and fish is a feasible way to lower the omega–6/omega–3 ratio.

The Israeli Paradox

Based upon adipose tissue analysis, LA intake in Israel has increased in recent years and was estimated to be approximately 12% of energy intake [6]. Recent data from Jerusalem suggested that an average of 10% is about the current intake [42]. Ninety percent of subjects in this study consumed more than 6% PUFA, and a quarter consumed more than 12% PUFA, of total energy intake. The P/S ratio was 0.9 on average, with a quarter of subjects reaching a value of 1.2 and above. This proportion of PUFA intake in Israel is very high, resulting in what is possibly the highest adipose content of LA in the world, around 25% (references in [6]). The recommended LA intake by an international workshop on the subject is 3% [21], while that of a British Nutrition Foundation task force is 6%, with a 'safe range' of 3–10% [43]; a report prepared for the Food and Drug Administration recommended that LA constitute 4–7% of total energy [2]. Until recently, the World Health Organization recommended PUFA comprising between 3 and 7% of total energy intake [44]; the study group stated then that this upper limit was set as '…existing population average intakes seldom exceeded 7% of energy…'. These data position Israel as a country with one of the highest levels of LA consumption in the world, probably due to the high LA content of the marketed oils in the country. Soy bean oil is the most common oil produced and consumed in Israel, accounting for over 85% of vegetable oils in the market [45]. Its LA content is about 50%, and its ALA content is about 7%.

With the establishment of the State of Israel and the arrival of many groups of immigrants, oil and fat intake rose from 15 kg/year/capita in 1950 to 21 kg/year/capita in 1970 [45]. In concert, fish intake dropped from 17 kg/year/capita in 1950, to 10 kg/year/capita in 1973. Current data from the Negev Nutritional Studies suggest that fish consumption in this relatively dry part of the country approximates only 3.6 kg/year/person [unpubl. obs.]. Hence, the omega–6/omega–3 ratio in Israel has been rising slowly for many years.

The dietary omega–6/omega–3 ratio in Europe has been estimated at 10–14:1 [6]. This ratio in the nutrition of British men was around 10:1 in 1980 and 8:1 in 1992, but adipose tissue analysis, which reflects long term actual consumption, suggested a practical ratio of 16:1 [46]. In Japan, this ratio approximates 4:1, due to both a low fat diet and a relatively high consumption of fish and ALA-containing vegetable oils [47]. In contrast to these regions of the world, Israelis are estimated to consume a much higher dietary omega–6/omega–3 ratio – about 22–26:1 [6]. Yet all these figures are far from a recommendation of 2:1 suggested by Okuyama et al. [9] for industrialized countries. This ratio is based on the observed increase in cancer, allergy and atherosclerotic disease in Japan, related, at least in part, to an increase in the omega–6/omega–3 ratio from 2.8:1 to 4:1 in the past 40 years.

The total amount of energy consumed in Israel during the late 1980s was lower than that of the USA and European countries except Sweden [3]. Data from the Israeli Central Bureau of Statistics showed that in 1992–1994, the average energy intake in Israel was about 3,100 kcal/day/capita, compared with about 3,300 kcal/day/capita in the Netherlands, 3,600 kcal/day/capita in the USA, and 3,700 kcal/day/capita in Belgium [4]. Similar relations were found for total fat intake, and all western countries consumed more total fat: about 120 g/day/capita in Israel, but 140 g/day/capita in UK, France and Italy, 150 g/day/capita in Canada, Spain and Greece, and 160 g/day/capita in the US [3]. Though a Mediterranean country, olive oil consumption in modern Israel is quite low, probably because of price constraints. In contrast to other western countries, animal fat intake is lower than that of vegetable oil – a supposedly positive nutritional choice. For example, butter consumption in Israel in the mid 1990s was the lowest among 20 countries worldwide [3].

Taken as a whole, the Israeli diet, low in total energy, total and animal fat, combined with high levels of cholesterol-lowering PUFA, seems a solid recipe for good health. Therefore, in Israel, a low prevalence of CAD and other dietary fat-related diseases, like diabetes and several types of cancer, may be anticipated.

Yet the prevalence of CAD, diabetes mellitus and cancer in Israel is comparable with other western countries. In Israel of 1995, the standardized mortality rate from CAD was 235 (males) and 168 (females) compared with 246 (males) and 131 (females) in the US and Europe [5]. The prevalence of diabetes mellitus in Israeli Jews in 1996 was 3.4%, compared with 5.4% of US citizens of the same year [48], yet the rate of deaths from diabetes mellitus in Israel ranked first worldwide [3]. The incidence of colorectal cancer was similar to that in the UK, Canada, Italy, and US whites [3]. Compared with the non-Jewish population of Israel, which have a more traditional diet, Jews have a much higher incidence of most types of cancer [5, 6]. Therefore, the theoretically promising nutrition profile in Israel does not translate to less morbidity. This is termed the Israeli Paradox, as it appears that high omega–6 intake, along with a high omega–6/omega–3 ratio, counteract the expected health benefits of the other components of the Israeli diet.

Lowering the Omega–6/Omega–3 Ratio Despite High LA Intake

Studies of omega–3 supplementation proved it could lower CAD and its risk factors in the general population. But can the high background LA intake be overcome with increasing omega–3 intake? Can the Israeli paradox be modified? Several studies in animals and man suggest that this may be possible in animals and man.

Adding fish oil to the diet of rats with dietary fat induced hyperinsulinemia can prevent the development of insulin resistance [49]. A cross-over study among hyperlipidemic subjects in Israel showed that ingestion of 15 g fish oil/day (=5.2 g of omega–3 PUFA) reduced triglyceride levels by 40% within 2 weeks of treatment [50]. This was accompanied by a 12% increase in HDL levels, without affecting total or LDL cholesterol levels. Serum, platelet and erythrocyte levels of omega–3 fatty acids were elevated, while the levels of LA and AA in erythrocytes were reduced. In another study, omega–3 supplementation was given to 48 hyperlipidemic, statin-treated CAD patients in Israel. This resulted in a reduction in CAD risk factors [51]. Compared with an olive-oil control group, there was a decrease in both total and LDL cholesterol, in triglyceride and in insulin levels. Here, the omega–3 fatty acids were offered in the form of a spread. In another study population – one with high LA intake (mean 7.5%) and a baseline LA:ALA ratio of about 17, increasing ALA intake and its levels in plasma cholesteryl-ester were associated with a decrease in blood pressure, but an increase in plasma triglycerides [52]. Yet in this study, even the subjects in the highest quintile of plasma ALA had high dietary LA:ALA ratios of 12.4. This point reinforces the fact that high background LA consumption can possibly mask the health benefits associated with ALA alone.

Future Research

While the optimal omega–6/omega–3 ratio is still not known, future research is needed. Large interventional studies with varying intake ratios would definitely be helpful but probably financially impossible to perform. A recent study from Israel correlated adipose tissue fatty acids, a measure of long term fatty acid intake, with acute myocardial infarction [42]. Here, tissue LA, tissue ALA, or the ratios between omega–6/omega–3 in adipose tissue, did not differ between subjects with myocardial infarctions and controls. However, AA levels were significantly higher in the cases. Interestingly, dietary PUFA amounts correlated well with tissue LA – but not with its metabolic end-product, AA. Hence, the path of dietary fat-adipose fat-CAD should be further elucidated. While the adipose tissue analyses are believed to be a true and objective reflection of dietary fat intake [53, 54], these results suggest that methods to assess the optimal dietary omega–6/omega–3 ratio should incorporate tissue analysis as well.

References

1 Keys A, Parlin RW: Serum cholesterol response to changes in dietary lipids. Am J Clin Nutr 1966;19:175–181.
2 Grundy AM: Evaluation of Publicly Available Scientific Evidence Regarding Certain Nutrient-Disease Relationships: Lipids and Cardiovascular Disease Bethesda. Life Sciences Research Office, Federation of American Societies for Experimental Biology, 1991.
3 Australian Institute of Health and Welfare: International health – how Australia compares. AIHW cat No PHE 8. Canberra, AIHW, 1998. Available at http://www.aihw.gov.au/publications/health/ihhac, accessed Sept 25, 2002.
4 Israeli Central Bureau of Statistics: 1999 Food balance sheet. Available at http://www.cbs.gov.il/hodaot2000/19_00_237.htm, accessed Sept 25, 2002.
5 Israel Ministry of Health web site, http://www.health.gov.il/units/healthisrael/63.htm, and http://www.health.gov.il/units/healthisrael/62.htm, accessed Sept 4, 2002.
6 Yam D, Eliraz A, Berry EM: Diet and disease – the Israeli paradox: possible dangers of a high omega–6 polyunsaturated fatty acid diet. Isr J Med Sci 1996;32:1134–1143.
7 Berry EM: Are diets high in omega 6 polyunsaturated fatty acids unhealthy? Eur Heart J Supplements 2001;39(suppl D):D37–D41.
8 Berry EM: Who's afraid of n-6 polyunsaturated fatty acids? Methodological considerations for assessing whether they are harmful. Nut Met Cardiovasc Dis 2001;11:181–188.
9 Okuyama H, Kobayashi T, Watanabe S: Dietary fatty acids – the n-6/n-3 balance and chronic elderly diseases: Excess linoleic acid and relative n-3 deficiency syndrome seen in Japan. Prog Lipid Res 1997;35:409–457.

10   Dewailly E, Blanchet C, Lemieux S, Sauve L, Gingras S, Ayotte P, Holub BJ: n-3 fatty acids and cardiovascular disease risk factors among the Inuit of Nunavik. Am J Clin Nutr 2001;74: 464–473.

11   Albert CM, Campos H, Stampfer MJ, Ridker PM, Manson JE, Willet WC, Ma J: Blood levels of long-chain n–3 fatty acids and the risk of sudden death. N Engl J Med 2002;346:1113–1118.

12   Hu FB, Bronner L, Willett WC, Stampfer MJ, Rexrode KM, Albert CM, Hunter D, Manson JE: Fish and omega 3 fatty acid intake and risk of coronary heart disease in women. JAMA 2002;287: 1815–1821.

13   Albert CM, Gaziano JM, Willett WC, Manson JE: Nut consumption and decreased risk of sudden cardiac death in the Physicians' Health Study. Arch Intern Med 2002;162:1382–1387.

14   Hu FB, Stampfer MJ, Manson JE, Rimm EB, Colditz GA, Rosner BA, Speizer FE, Hennekens CH, Willet WC: Frequent nut consumption and risk of coronary heart disease in women: prospective cohort study. BMJ 1998;317:1341–1345.

15   Hu FB, Stampfer MJ, Manson JE, Rimm EB, Wolk A, Colditz GA, Hennekens CH, Willett WC: Dietary intake of alpha-linolenic acid and risk of ischemic heart disease among women. Am J Clin Nutr 1999;69:890–897.

16   De Lorgeril M, Salen P, Martin J-L, Monjaud I, Delaye J, Mamelle N: Mediterranean diet, traditional risk factors, and the rate of cardiovascular complications after myocardial infarction: Final report of the Lyon Diet Heart Study. Circulation 1999;99:779–785.

17   GISSI-Prevenzione Investigators: Dietary supplementation with n-3 polyunsaturated fatty acids and vitamin E after myocardial infarction: results of the GISSI-Prevenzione trial. Lancet 1999; 354:447–455.

18   Singh RB, Dubnov G, Niaz MA, Saraswati Ghosh, Singh R, Rastogi SS, Manor O, Pella D, Berry EM: Effect of an Indo-Mediterranean diet on progression of coronary artery disease in high risk patients (Indo-Mediterranean Diet Heart Study): A randomised single-blind trial. Lancet 2002;360:1455–1461.

19   Bucher HC, Hengstler P, Schindler C, Meier G: N-3 polyunsaturated fatty acids in coronary heart disease: A meta-analysis of randomized controlled trials. Am J Med 2002;112:298–304.

20   de Deckere EAM, Korver O, Verschuren PM, Katan MB: Health aspects of fish and n-3 polyunsaturated fatty acids from plant and marine origin. Eur J Clin Nutr 1998;52:749–753.

21   Simopoulos AP, Leaf A, Salem N: Essentiality of and recommended dietary intakes for omega–6 and omega–3 fatty acids. Ann Nutr Metab 1999;43:127–130.

22   Rustan AC, Nenseter MS, Drevon CA: Omega 3 and omega 6 fatty acids in the insulin resistance syndrome. Ann NY Acad Sci 1997;827:310–326.

23   Djousse L, Pankow JS, Eckfeldt JH, Folsom AR, Hopkins PN, Province MA, Hong Y, Ellison RC: Relation between dietary linolenic acid and coronary artery disease in the National Heart, Lung, and Blood Institute Family Heart Study. Am J Clin Nutr 2001;74:612–619.

24   Iso H, Sato S, Umemura U, Kudo M, Koike K, Kitamura A, Imano H, Okamura T, Naito Y, Shimamoto T: Linoleic acid, other fatty acids, and the risk of stroke. Stroke 2002;33:2086–2093.

25   Berry EM, Kohen R: Is the biological antioxidant system integrated and regulated? Med Hypotheses 1999;53:397–401.

26   Machlin LJ: Effect of dietary linolenate on the proportion of linoleate and arachidonate in liver fat. Nature 1962;194:868–870.

27   Mohrhauer H, Holman RT: Effect of linolenic acid upon the metabolism of linoleic acid. J Nutr 1963;81:67–74.

28   Iso H, Rexrode KM, Stampfer MJ, Manson JE, Colditz GA, Speizer FE, Hennekens CH, Willet WC: Intake of fish and omega 3 fatty acids and risk of stroke in women. JAMA 2001;285: 304–312.

29   Krauss RM, Eckel RH, Howard B, Appel LJ, Daniels SR, Deckelbaum RJ, Erdman JW Jr, Kris-Etherton P, Goldberg IJ, Kotchen TA, Lichtenstein AH, Mitch WE, Mullis R, Robinson K, Wylie-Rosett J, St Jeor S, Suttie J, Tribble DL, Bazzarre TL: AHA dietary guidelines: revision 2000: A statement for healthcare professionals from the Nutrition Committee of the American Heart Association. Circulation 2000;102:2284–2299.

30   Capone SL, Bagga D, Glaspi JA: Relationship between omega–6 and omega–3 fatty acid ratios and breast cancer (editorial). Nutrition 1997;13:822–824.

31   Maillard V, Bougnoux P, Ferrari P, Jourdan ML, Pinault M, Lavillionnaire F, Body G, Le Flotch O, Chajes V: n-3 and n-6 fatty acids in breast adipose tissue and relative risk of breast cancer in a case-control study in Tours, France. Int J Cancer 2002;98:78–83.

32   Simopoulos AP: The Mediterranean diets: What is so special about the diet of Greece? The scientific evidence. J Nutr 2001;131:3065S–3073S.

33   Albertazzi P, Coupland K: Polyunsaturated fatty acids: Is there a role in postmenopausal osteoporosis prevention. Maturitas 2002;42:13–22.

34   Vanpapendorp DH, Coetzer H, Kruger MG: Biochemical profile of osteoporotic patients on essential fatty-acids supplementation. Nutr Res 1995;15:325–334.

35   Kruger MC, Coetzer H, de Winter R, Gerike G, van Papendorp DH: Calcium, gamma-linolenic acid and eicosopentaenoic acid supplementation in senile osteoporosis. Aging Clin Exp Res 1998; 10:385–394.

36   Bassey EJ, Lettlewood JE, Rthwell MC, Pye DW: Lack of effects of supplementation with essential fatty acids on bone mineral density in healthy pre and post menopausal women: Two randomized controlled trial of Efacal vs calcium alone. Br J Nutr 2000;83:629–635.

37   Simopoulos AP: Essential fatty acids in health and chronic disease. Am J Clin Nutr 1999; 70(suppl):560s–569s.

38   Eaton SB, Eaton SB III, Sinclair AJ, Cordain L, Mann NJ: Dietary intake of long-chain polyunsaturated fatty acids during the Paleolithic. Wld Rev Nutr Diet. Basel, Karger, 1998, vol 83, pp 12–23.

39   World Health Organization: Fats and oils in human nutrition: Report of a joint expert consultation. Food and Agriculture Organization of the United Nations and the World Health Organization. FAO Food Nutr Pap 1995;57:1–147.

40   World Health Organization: Diet, nutrition, and the prevention of chronic diseases. Tech Report No. 916, 2003.

41   Feldman EB: The scientific evidence for a beneficial health relationship between walnuts and coronary heart disease. J Nutr 2002;132:1062S–1101S.

42   Kark JD, Kaufmann NA, Binka F, Goldberger N, Berry EM: Adipose tissue n-6 fatty acids and acute myocardial infarction in a population consuming a diet high in polyunsaturated fatty acids. Am J Clin Nutr 2003;77:796–802.

43   The British Nutrition Foundation: Unsaturated fatty acids. Nutritional and physiological significance. The Report of the British Nutrition Foundation's Task Force. London, Chapman & Hill, 1992.

44   World Health Organization: Diet, nutrition, and the prevention of chronic diseases. Tech Report No 797, 1990.

45   Guggenheim K, Kaufmann NA: Nutritional health in a changing society – studies from Israel. World Rev Nutr Diet. Basel, Karger, 1976, vol 2, pp 217–240.

46   Sanders TAB: Polyunsaturated fatty acids in the food chain in Europe. Am J Clin Nutr 2000; 71(suppl):176S–178S.

47   Sugano M, Hirahara F: Polyunsaturated fatty acids in the food chain in Japan. Am J Clin Nutr 2000;71:189–196.

48   Mokdad A, Ford ES, Bowman BA, Nelson DE, Engelgau MM, Vinicor F, Marks JS: Diabetes Trends in the US: 1990–1998. Diabetes Care 2000;23:1278–1283.

49   Storfien LH, Kraegen EW, Chisholm DJ: Fish oil prevents insulin resistance induced by high fat feeding in rats. Science 1987;237:885–888.

50   Green P, Fuchs J, Schoenfeld N, Leibovici L, Lurie Y, Beigel Y, Rotenberg Z, Mamet R, Budowski P: Effects of fish-oil ingestion on cardiovascular risk factors in hyperlipidemic subjects in Israel: A randomized, double-blind crossover study. Am J Clin Nutr 1990;52:1118–1124.

51   Yam D, Bott-Kanner G, Genin I, Shinitzky M, Klainman E: The effect of omega–3 fatty acids on risk factors for cardiovascular diseases (in Hebrew). Harefuah 2001;140:1156–1158.

52   Bemelmans WJE, Muskiet FAJ, Feskens EJM, de Vries JHM, Broer J, May JF, Meyboom-de Jong B: Associations of alpha-linolenic acid and linoleic acid with risk factors for coronary heart disease. Eur J Clin Nutr 2000;54:865–871.

53   Van Staveren WA, Deurenberg P, Katan MB, Burema J, de Groot LC, Hoffmans MD: Validity of the fatty acid composition of subcutaneous fat tissue microbiopsies as an estimate of the long-term

average fatty acid composition of the diet of separate individuals. Am J Epidemiol 1986;123: 455–463.

54   Hunter DJ, Rimm EB, Sacks FM, Stampfer MJ, Colditz GA, Litin LB, Willet WC: Comparison of measures of fatty acid intake by subcutaneous fat aspirate, food frequency questionnaire, and diet records in a free-living population of US men. Am J Epidemiol 1992;135:418–427.

Prof. Elliot M. Berry, MD
Department of Human Nutrition and Metabolism
Hebrew University–Hadassah Medical School
Jerusalem, 91120 (Israel)
Tel. +972 2 6758298, Fax +972 2 6431105, E-Mail berry@md.huji.ac.il

Simopoulos AP, Cleland LG (eds): Omega–6/Omega–3 Essential Fatty Acid Ratio:
The Scientific Evidence. World Rev Nutr Diet. Basel, Karger, 2003, vol 92, pp 92–108

....

Linoleic Acid to Alpha-Linolenic Acid Ratio

From Clinical Trials to Inflammatory Markers of Coronary Artery Disease

*Antonis Zampelas[a], George Paschos[a], Loukianos Rallidis[b],
Nikos Yiannakouris[c]*

[a] Department of Nutrition and Dietetics, Harokopio University, Athens,
[b] Department of Cardiology, General Hospital of Nikea, Piraeus, and
[c] Department of Home Economics and Ecology, Harokopio University, Athens, Greece

The antiatherogenic effect of the very long-chain ω3 fatty acids, namely eicosapentaenoic (EPA, 20:5ω3) and docosahexaenoic (DHA, 22:6ω3) acids has been well documented [1–4]. However, although fatty fish is the richest source of these fatty acids, its consumption is low in Western societies [5–7]. Lately, research has been focused on the effects of α-linolenic acid (ALA, 18:3ω3), the precursor of EPA and DHA, on parameters which affect the process of atherogenesis. A number of issues have been considered: (1) which parameters of the lipoprotein metabolism, the blood homeostasis, the endothelial function, and the immune and inflammatory response are influenced by increased ALA intake; (2) what is the rate of conversion of ALA to EPA and DHA; (3) how important is the ratio of linoleic acid (LA, 18:2ω6):ALA in order to establish an optimum intake of ALA and maximize its beneficial effects. The results so far are rather conflicting depending on the study design and in particular the dose and the duration of the study, the comparisons that have been made (i.e. ALA vs. LA, ALA vs. EPA/DHA, etc.), and the subjects involved (healthy volunteers, hyperlipidemics, coronary heart disease patients). It is also noteworthy that although it is known that high intake of LA decreases the conversion of ALA to EPA and DHA [8–11], studies examining the effects of LA:ALA ratio on the risk of coronary artery disease (CAD), especially parameters of the inflammatory response are only a few.

Inflammation Markers and Risk of Coronary Artery Disease

It is well documented that inflammation plays a central role in athero-sclerosis since all stages of atherosclerosis are characterized by the dynamic interaction of inflammatory cells, cytokines and chemokines in the arterial wall [12]. The conventional risk factors (atherogenic lipoproteins, cigarette smoking, hyperglycemia, hypertension) seem to be the main injurious factors that initiate and promote the atherogenic process by triggering the inflammatory reaction.

The earliest detectable cellular event in atherosclerosis involves the attachment of monocytes to endothelial cells. This inflammatory response is facilitated by leukocyte adhesion molecules, expressed on the surface of endothelial cells, under the direction of proinflammatory cytokines such as interleukin-1 (IL-1) and tumor necrosis factor-α (TNF-α). Subsequent migration of monocytes into the subendothelial space is promoted by the chemoattractant cytokine, monocyte chemoattractant protein-1, which is produced by the endothelium in response mainly to oxidized low-density lipoprotein (LDL). The monocytes into the subendothelium are transformed into macrophages that accumulate modified LDL particles and become foam cells, the hallmark of fatty streaks. Further injurious stimuli may continue the attraction and accumulation of macrophages, and activated T lymphocytes and the smooth muscle proliferation within the growing atherosclerotic lesion. Macrophages also contribute to plaque vulnerability by production of metalloproteinases that break collagen and weaken the fibrous plaque cap. The expression of metalloproteinases is induced by pro-inflammatory cytokines. Cytokines can also trigger apoptosis of smooth muscle cells contributing to the weakening of the fibrous cap and making it prone to rupture. The disruption of the atherosclerotic plaque with the subsequent thrombosis leads to coronary events [13].

In view of the persuasive evidence implicating inflammation in athero-thrombosis, not surprisingly many circulating markers of inflammation strongly correlate with coronary events, including unstable angina, myocardial infarction and death. Among these markers special attention has been focused on C-reactive protein (CRP), serum amyloid A (SAA), IL-6, TNF-α, macrophage colony stimulating factor (MCSF) and a number of leukocyte adhesion molecules [14].

CRP is the best-studied inflammatory marker [15]. It is an acute-phase reactant produced by the liver in response to IL-6 and it predicts coronary events and coronary mortality in the primary and secondary prevention of coronary artery disease [15, 16]. In normal healthy individuals, CRP is a long-term predictor of coronary artery disease, within a range which previously was considered to be normal. A meta-analysis of prospective population-based studies has shown an approximately 2-fold increase in relative risk for major coronary events in individuals at the upper tertile of CRP compared with those in the lower tertile [17]. In the setting of stable coronary artery disease, CRP levels >3 mg/l is a long-term predictor of cardiac events while in acute coronary syndromes a level >10 mg/l has a better predictive value. Importantly, the predictive value of CRP adds to the information provided by the classic risk factors, while in acute coronary syndromes are independent of troponins. There are also findings suggesting an active role of CRP in the atherosclerotic process [16, 18]. CRP has been found in atherosclerotic lesions and CRP-opsonised native LDL-cholesterol by macrophages seems to contribute to foam cell formation. In addition, CRP can activate complement in atherosclerotic plaques leading to plaque instability, can stimulate tissue factor production by macrophages promoting coagulation and can induce expression of cellular adhesion molecules.

Other inflammatory markers that have also been studied, although less extensively, are IL-6, SAA, TNF-α, MCSF and soluble forms of cellular adhesion molecules. There are studies indicating the prognostic value of these markers in the setting of primary and secondary prevention of CAD. However, the lack of reliable and reproducible assays limits the use of these markers to the research setting [15]. Cytokines, such as TNF-α and IL-1β are involved in the acute-phase protein synthesis but only IL-6 can stimulate synthesis of all acute-phase proteins involved in the inflammatory response namely, CRP, SAA, fibrinogen and others [19]. IL-6 is synthesized in the subcutaneous adipose tissue and in cells of the immune system [20], correlates with body mass index (BMI) and percent body fat and it is suggested that it may be a link between obesity and insulin resistance [21]. TNF-α and IL-1 are synthesized in the monocytes and macrophages. Production of TNF-α, IL-1 and IL-6 may be beneficial in response to infection, but overproduction, which may occur as a result of an inflammatory response, may have pathological implications [22].

Recently, it has been suggested that, in clinical practice, CRP (hs-CRP) can be used as an adjunct to the major risk factors, to further assess the absolute risk of individuals without established CAD, and particularly in those with an intermediate (10–20% risk in 10 years) [23]. The recommended cut-off-points are: CRP >3 mg/l (high risk), 1–3 mg/l (average risk) and <1 mg/l (low risk). The presence of elevated hs-CRP levels in these individuals will probably lead to intensification of medical treatment or will motivate them to improve their lifestyle.

Epidemiological and Clinical Trials

Epidemiological studies suggest that ALA may have a beneficial effect in decreasing the risk of CAD but this evidence remains inconclusive. In the

EURAMIC Study [23], a relative risk for myocardial infarction (MI) of 0.42 was found when the highest quintile of adipose tissue ALA was compared to the lowest in patients with first MI (n = 639) and controls (n = 700). However, the protective effect of ALA lost its significance after adjusting for classic risk factors (mainly smoking). A protective effect of DHA was not detected.

In the National Heart, Lung and Blood Institute Family Heart Study, 4,584 participants were allocated to five quintiles, according to dietary ALA intake [24]. The ALA intake varied from a mean of 0.53–1.14 g per day for the men and from 0.46 to 0.96 g per day for the women. The results of this epidemiological study indicated that there was an inverse association between ALA intake and the prevalence of odds ratio of CAD. In addition, participants in the highest quintile of both ALA and LA intakes had 56% lower prevalence odds ratio of CAD than did the participants in the lowest quintile of both fatty acid intakes. In accordance with this study, in the Nurses Health Study [25] and in the all-male Health Professionals Study [26], a dose-response relationship was observed between ALA intake and relative risk of fatal ischemic heart disease. Especially, in the Nurses Health Study after adjustment for age, standard coronary risk factors and dietary intake of LA, ALA was associated with a lower relative risk of fatal ischemic heart disease (from the lowest to the highest quintiles the relative risk was 1.00, 0.99, 0.90, 0.67, and 0.55 (p for trend = 0.01)). In the Health Professionals Study, the intake of ALA was inversely associated with the risk of myocardial infarction. This association became significant after adjustment for non-dietary risk factors and was strengthened after adjustment for total fat intake (relative risk 0.41 for 1% increase in energy, p for trend <0.01). However, in the Zutphen Elderly Study, ALA was not found to be beneficially associated with 10-year risk of coronary artery disease incidence [27]. In this study, the authors divided the subjects in three quintiles according to the dietary ALA intake but failed to show any significant association with CAD risk. The authors speculated that there may be an association between ALA and trans fatty acid intakes. Even though the LA:ALA ratio was not taken into consideration in this study, it could be roughly estimated that in all the quintiles it was approaching 10:1. This may have also complicated any association, given the fact that in order to observe any effect of ALA, LA intake must also be relatively low.

Regarding clinical trials, even though research looking at the effects of either ω6 or ω3 fatty acids on cardiovascular risk factors began in the middle of the last century, there are only a few clinical trials investigating the effects of these fatty acids and especially the ω3 fatty acids, on end points of the disease, and none of them was designed to look at the ratio of ω6 to ω3 fatty acids, except the Lyon Diet Heart Study that consisted of a dietary pattern based on a modified diet of Crete and a ratio of LA:ALA of 4:1 [28]. This was a major trial

Table 1. Design and major outcomes of clinical trials

Study	Number of subjects	LA:ALA ratio	Duration years	Cholesterol levels	Outcome
Lyon Diet Heart Study	605	4:1	5	unchanged	65% decrease in CAD mortality in post-MI patients on a Mediterranean-type diet enriched with ALA.
Indo-Mediterranean Diet Heart Study	499 (intervention) 509 (control)	9:1	2	decreased	fewer total cardiac endpoints in the intervention group than in controls (39 vs. 76 events): reduced sudden cardiac deaths (6 vs. 16) and non-fatal MI (21 vs. 43).
Indian Experiment of Infarct Survival Study	122 (EPA) 122 (ALA)		1	modest decrease	24.5 and 28% decrease in the cardiac events in the EPA and ALA groups, respectively: the decrease in blood lipoproteins was not the cause of the benefit
MARGARIN Study	280	varied from 3.9 to 27.7	2	NS compared to control	no difference between the ALA and LA groups in the 10-year estimated ischemic heart disease risk.

looking at the effects of the modified diet of Crete, high in ALA, on the rate of recurrence following a first MI. In the modified diet of the Crete Group (experimental group), combining either cardiac death and nonfatal MI was reduced as well as cardiac death plus major secondary end points (unstable angina, stroke, heart failure, pulmonary or peripheral embolism) and cardiac death plus minor events requiring hospital admission, compared to the prudent American Heart Association Step I diet group (table 1). In the intervention group, the ω6:ω3 ratio was 4:1 but, in addition, total fat and saturated fat as well as cholesterol intakes were lower and dietary fiber intake was higher than in the control group. Thus, although the results are striking and the magnitude of the effect of the diet on the disease end points could be comparable to drug treatment, or even more, they cannot be solely attributed to an increase in ALA intake.

In another secondary prevention trial, the Indo-Mediterranean Diet Heart Study, 499 patients were allocated to a diet rich in whole grains, fruits, vegetables, walnuts and almonds and 501 controls consumed a diet similar to the National Cholesterol Education Program (NCEP) Step I Diet [29]. The ALA intake in the intervention group was estimated to be 1.8 g daily compared to 0.8 in the control group. The results of the study showed that total cardiac end points were fewer in the intervention group than in the control group. These changes could be partly attributed to the increase in ALA intakes and the ω6:ω3 ratio in the intervention group was 9.1:1 compared to 21:1 in the control group. However, other dietary parameters, such as dietary fat, cholesterol and fiber intakes were also altered and therefore caution should be also made in the interpretation of the results and the magnitude of the effect of ALA on the outcome of the trial.

In the Indian Experiment of Infarct Survival Study [30], 112 patients were given 1.08 g/day EPA, 120 patients were given 2.9 g/day and 118 patients were the placebo group. After 1 year of treatment, total cardiac events and non-fatal infarctions were significantly less in the 2 experimental groups compared with the placebo group. However, reductions in blood lipoproteins in the 2 experimental groups were modest and did not appear to be the cause of the benefit.

The Mediterranean Alpha-linolenic Enriched Groningen Dietary Intervention (MARGARIN) study was partly designed to look at the effects of ALA on cardiovascular risk factors and to estimate the risk of ischemic heart disease (IHD) at 2 years in patients with multiple cardiovascular risk factors [31]. Interestingly, at the end of the study, the ALA group had similar 10-year estimated IHD risk as the LA group even though it had also a higher ratio of total to HDL cholesterol, higher plasma triglycerides but lower plasma fibrinogen levels. At the end of the period studied LA:ALA ratios in the ALA groups varied from 3.9:1.0 and 4.5:1.0 in women, and from 4.2 to 15.1 in men, according to the interventions (with or without nutritional education, respectively).

It is therefore considered necessary to design a clinical trial examining the effects of the ratio of LA to ALA on CAD disease end-points by keeping other dietary parameters constant.

Metabolic Studies

As previously mentioned, evidence from epidemiological studies and large clinical trials is not conclusive regarding the exact magnitude of the effect of ALA and LA:ALA ratio on risk for CAD. In addition, there is a suggestion that ALA does not have a major effect on coagulation and fibrinolysis [32, 33] and even in the CARDIA Study, ω3 fatty acids from fish oils did not affect hemostatic factors [34], whereas they had beneficial effects in older adults [35]. However, in a study by Renaud et al. [36] it was observed that ALA intake may have anti-aggregatory properties since it was inversely correlated with some platelet functions. Regarding the effects on blood lipids, there is evidence which suggests that replacing LA by ALA in healthy adults has no further effects [37, 38] and that ALA does not have the hypotriglyceridemic effect of high EPA/DHA diets [39]. However, it has also been suggested that ALA lowers cholesterol levels when it replaces saturated fat in the diet [40].

Over the years there has been great interest in the effects of the different types of dietary fatty acids on several parameters of the immune system. This is partly because the long-chain ω6 polyunsaturated fatty acid (PUFA) arachidonic acid is the precursor of 2-series prostaglandins and 4-series leukotrienes, which have potent roles in regulating inflammatory and immune responses [39, 41]. Comparisons of the in vitro effects of different fatty acids on lymphocyte function were first carried out about 25 years ago and it was observed that LA and arachidonic acid were both potent inhibitors of mitogen-stimulated proliferation of rodent [42] and human lymphocytes [43–45], with arachidonic acid being the most potent. Later studies showed that the ω3 PUFAs, ALA, EPA and DHA, were also potent inhibitors of the mitogen-stimulated proliferation of rodent [46–48] and human lymphocytes [49–52]. The role of ALA in modulating immune mechanisms, namely suppression of T-cell responses, has been predominantly studied in animals [53–58]. There is only a limited number of human studies on the effect of dietary ALA on immune system function and on markers of inflammatory response [59, 60, 62, 64].

The first study that showed a significant decrease in human blood lymphocyte proliferation, after following a flaxseed oil diet for 6 weeks, was carried out by Kelley et al. [59]. Ten healthy free-living young men participated in this study. The subjects consumed all meals at the Western Human Nutrition Research Center. There was a stabilization period of 14 days at the start when the subjects consumed a baseline diet. The ratio of LA:ALA in the baseline diet was 23.9:1.0. Five subjects consumed a flaxseed oil supplemented diet and the ratio of LA:ALA was significantly decreased to 0.7:1.0. The dramatic change in the ratio of LA:ALA, after introducing subjects to the flaxseed oil diet, resulted in a significant suppression of the peripheral blood mononuclear cell proliferation, when cells were cultured with T-cell mitogens (table 2). A second result was the suppression in the delayed hypersensitivity skin response to seven recall antigens. Taken together, the results of this study suggested that

Table 2. Relationship between LA:ALA ratio in the diet and markers of inflammatory response in humans

Study	Number of subjects	ALA intake/day g	LA:ALA ratio	Experimental period weeks	Effects
Kelley et al. [59]	5	21.2	0.7:1.0	6	↓ lymphocyte proliferation
Caughey et al. [60]	15	13.7	0.6:1.0	4	↓ TNF-α, IL-1β production by monocytes
Thies et al. [62]	8	2.0	3.5:1.0	12	no effect on lymphocyte proliferation, cytokine production
Rallidis et al. [64]	50	8.1	1.3:1.0	12	↓ CRP, SAA, IL-6

changing the LA:ALA ratio to lower than 1:1 could result in a suppression of some of the indices of cell-mediated immunity.

In a later study, Caughey et al. [60] designed a parallel case-control study to test the effect of ω3 fatty acids from vegetable and fish oils on TNF-α, IL-1β and the production by human monocytes. Thirty healthy male subjects aged 24–44 years were selected to participate in the study. Fifteen of the participants were given flaxseed oil supplements providing 13.7 g/day of ALA for 4 weeks, which resulted in a LA:ALA ratio of 0.6:1.0. The increase in dietary ALA resulted in the increase of cellular concentrations of ALA and its metabolite EPA by 3.0- and 2.3-fold, respectively. After 4 weeks of the experimental period, TNF-α, IL-1β, thromboxane B_2 and prostaglandin E_2 production by human monocytes decreased by 30, 31, 29 and 30%, respectively. Mononuclear cellular EPA concentrations were found to be significantly and inversely correlated with both TNF-α and IL-1β production. In this study, an important determinant of the efficiency with which dietary ALA elevated cellular EPA was the amount of dietary LA. It has been shown that the ratio of dietary ALA to LA has a much greater positive influence on the tissue concentrations of EPA than the absolute amount of dietary ALA [61].

Thies et al. [62], in a relatively recent study, investigated the effect of moderate supplementation with encapsulated oil blends rich in ALA, and other ω6 and ω3 polyunsaturated fatty acids, upon lymphocyte proliferation and cytokine production. Eight healthy, free-living subjects aged 55–75 years were supplemented with 2 g ALA per day for 12 weeks. The amount of ALA included in the supplement increased total ALA intake by 3-fold. Even so, the ratio of LA:ALA in the diet decreased from 11.0:1.0 to 3.5:1.0. ALA was absent from plasma phospholipids in most subjects at baseline and did not increase significantly after the ALA supplementation period. The products of

Table 3. Inflammatory markers before and after the intervention in the ALA and LA groups (values of inflammatory markers are expressed as median and 25th and 75th percentile)

Variables	At the beginning of the intervention	At the end of the intervention	p value
ALA group (n = 50)			
CRP, mg/l	1.24 (0.72–3.70)	0.93 (0.56–1.80)	0.0008
SAA, mg/l	3.24 (2.30–5.30)	2.39 (1.70–3.90)	0.0001
IL-6, pg/ml	2.18 (1.35–3.90)	1.70 (1.30–2.80)	0.01
LA group (n = 26)			
CRP, mg/l	1.54 (0.62–3.10)*	1.25 (0.64–1.70)	0.35
SAA, mg/l	3.52 (2.10–4.90)*	3.34 (2.15–4.40)	0.58
IL-6, pg/ml	1.77 (1.30–2.70)*	2.20 (1.10–2.70)	0.69

*p = NS compared to the corresponding levels in the ALA group.

ALA elongation and desaturation (EPA and DHA) were also not significantly elevated in plasma phospholipids. Thus, it appeared that ALA was not incorporated into plasma phospholipids in significant amounts after an increase in ALA intake by 3-fold, when the LA:ALA ratio was 3.5:1.0. Furthermore, if it was elongated and desaturated, the products of this process were not preferentially incorporated into plasma phospholipids. Supplementation with ALA was not found to significantly affect natural killer (NK) cell activity [63], mitogen-stimulated lymphocyte proliferation, or production of IL-2, or IFN-c by mononuclear cells [62]. The results of this study suggest that a moderate increase in ALA intake by healthy adults, changing LA:ALA ratio to 3.5:1.0, does not affect immunity and markers of inflammation.

However, results from a study carried out from our group [64], indicated that supplementing the diet of dyslipidemic patients with 8.1 g of ALA per day for 12 weeks and subsequently changing the ratio of LA:ALA from approximately 13.2:1.0 in the safflower oil supplemented group (n = 26) to 1.3:1.0 in the linseed oil supplemented group (n = 50), resulted in a decrease in serum concentrations of CRP, SAA and IL-6 (table 3). We also did not observe a change in blood cholesterol levels in the ALA group but there was a small decrease in HDL cholesterol. The reduction of the inflammatory markers in the ALA group was independent of lipid changes since there was no significant correlation between changes in inflammatory markers with those in lipids. Our results indicate that only a marked increase in ALA intake, resulting in a LA:ALA ratio of approximately 1:1, could induce anti-inflammatory and immunosuppressive effects in a relatively short-term period.

Genotypic Influences on the Response of Inflammatory Markers to ω3 Fatty Acids

As indicated above, it is quite possible that a high ratio of LA:ALA in the diet could limit the effectiveness of ALA as an anti-inflammatory agent. The discovery of single-nucleotide polymorphisms in the promoter regions of cytokine genes which influence the level of expression of the respective cytokines [65] is of particular interest because genetic variation could also influence responsiveness to ALA, at least in terms of cytokine suppression and the inflammatory response, and may explain why in some studies showing an anti-inflammatory effect of ω3 PUFAs, this effect is not demonstrable in all subjects [66].

In vivo studies have shown basal IL-6 levels to be twice as high in healthy subjects homozygous for the G allele of a common −174G/C polymorphism in the 5′ flanking region of the IL-6 gene than in those homozygous for the C allele [67]. Single nucleotide polymorphisms in the TNF-α and lymphotoxin-α (also known as TNF-β) genes influence the amount of TNF-α produced after an inflammatory stimulus [68] and appear to have clinical significance. For example, individuals who are homozygous for the TNF-α −308 (TNF2) allele or for the lymphotoxin-α +252 (TNFB2) allele show higher levels of TNF-α production and increased mortality in malaria infection and sepsis, respectively, compared to individuals heterozygous or homozygous for the more common TNF1 and TNFB1 alleles [69–71].

In a recent study, Grimble et al. [72] investigated the effects of the supplementation of 6 g fish oil/day (which provided 1.8 g ω3 PUFAs/day) for 12 weeks, on ex vivo TNF-α production by peripheral blood mononuclear cells in 111 young men, in relation to polymorphisms in the TNF-α and lymphotoxin-α genes. In this study, there was no information on dietary LA and ALA intakes, or the ratio of ω6:ω3 PUFAs, but a significant increase in the proportions of EPA and DHA in plasma phospholipids was observed at the end of the supplementation period. When data from all subjects were analyzed without any genetic component being considered, no significant effect of fish oil supplementation was found. However, sensitivity to fish oil supplementation was found to be influenced by pre-supplementation TNF-α production, with 86% of the subjects in the highest pre-supplementation tertile responding with a significant reduction in TNF-α production. In the highest tertile, mean production decreased significantly by 43%. Most importantly, a significant interaction was observed between TNF-α genotype and inherent TNF-α production in determining the extent of the decrease in TNF-α production that followed fish-oil supplementation, i.e. the decrease in TNF-α production among individuals in the highest tertile of pre-supplementation TNF-α production was significantly greater if subjects were carriers of the TNF2 allele than if they had the TNF1/TNF1 genotype. Moreover, in the lowest tertile of TNF-α production, only TNFB1/TNFB2 heterozygous subjects were responsive to the suppressive effect of fish oil. These data indicate that sensitivity to the anti-inflammatory effects of long-chain ω3 PUFAs is influenced by individual genotypic characteristics. No similar studies have explored the potential anti-inflammatory effects of ALA in relation to gene polymorphisms.

Interestingly, in a subsequent analysis of our data showing a beneficial effect of ALA on systemic markers of inflammation in dyslipidemic subjects [64], we found that the common apolipoprotein E (apo E) polymorphism influences responsiveness to this fatty acid. Specifically, we found that ALA supplementation (8.1 g/day for 12 weeks; LA:ALA ratio = 1.3:1.0) resulted in a significant reduction in the serum concentration of SAA and MCSF in subjects carrying the apo E3/E3 and E3/E4 genotypes, in addition to a significant reduction in CRP and IL-6 levels in E3/E3 individuals, but produced no effects on any of the inflammatory markers in the group of E2 allele carriers [unpubl. data]. The mechanism(s) underlying the above genotypic effects is at present unknown; however, apo E – which is best known for its role in the maintenance of plasma cholesterol levels – appears to be also directly involved in the regulation of chronic inflammatory responses [73], and thus our findings, if confirmed, may be of significance.

Further studies are necessary to examine the potential beneficial effects of ALA on inflammation in relation to a balanced ω6:ω3 ratio, which should also take into consideration genetic variation.

Discussion

Previous studies have shown that the effectiveness of dietary ALA on suppressing cytokine production depends on its conversion to EPA and DHA [60]. Because LA and ALA use the same enzymes for desaturation and elongation, the competition between ω6 and ω3 fatty acids provides a potential explanation for the importance of the LA:ALA ratio on the anti-inflammatory and immunosuppressive effectiveness of the dietary intervention that was observed in the studies mentioned above.

The mechanisms underlying the reduction of inflammatory markers levels following supplementation with ALA remain unknown. However, alteration in the type of arachidonic acid metabolites produced, on stimulation of mononuclear cells, may explain partly the decrease in cytokines production. Arachidonic acid is usually the principal precursor for eicosanoid synthesis since the membranes of most cells contain large amounts of arachidonic acid, compared with EPA [74]. Arachidonic acid in cell membranes can be mobilized by various phospholipase enzymes, most notably phospholipase A_2. The free arachidonic acid can subsequently act as a substrate for cyclooxygenase (COX), forming 2-series prostaglandins and related compounds, or for one of the three lipoxygenase (LOX) enzymes forming 4-series leukotrienes and related compounds. ALA, on the other hand, blocks the synthesis of arachidonic acid by LA, in an early step of the metabolic pathway, before EPA and DHA start competing with the $\omega 6$ fatty acids in the metabolic process. Since increased consumption of ALA results in a decrease in the amount of arachidonic acid in the membranes of inflammatory and immune cells, there will be less substrate available for synthesis of eicosanoids from arachidonic acid [75]. Furthermore, EPA competitively inhibits the oxygenation of arachidonic acid by COX. Thus, ALA supplementation results in a decreased capacity of immune cells to synthesize eicosanoids from arachidonic acid. In addition, EPA is able to act as a substrate for both COX and 5-LOX, giving rise to derivatives, which have a different structure and function from those, produced from arachidonic acid. The eicosanoids produced from EPA are often less biologically potent than the analogues synthesized from arachidonic acid (e.g. LTB_5 is only about 10% as potent as LTB_4 as a chemotactic agent and in promoting lysosomal enzyme release), although the full range of biological activities of these compounds has not been investigated [74]. It has been suggested that $\omega 3$ fatty acids lead to a suppression of thromboxane A2 (TXA2) synthesis in monocytes and this results in a decrease in TNF-α and IL-1β synthesis [76].

The evidence from clinical trials and metabolic studies suggest that increased intake of ALA can decrease the risk of CAD especially in the secondary prevention. There is also a limited number of studies which show that a low ratio of LA:ALA may decrease some inflammatory markers of CAD. Taking also into account that ALA may not have profound hypolipidemic effects, it may be suggested that its main mechanism of action could be through its effect on the inflammatory markers. EPA and DHA are considered potent anti-inflammatory agents and therefore the rate of conversion of ALA to EPA and DHA is of importance. This rate, though, is rather low because ALA is mainly oxidized. It has been suggested that for every 10 g of ALA, 0.5–1.0 g of EPA is incorporated to complex lipids [77] and that the conversion of ALA to DHA is very low or even absent in adults and in special groups such as infants, in some hypertensives, some diabetics and the elderly [8, 10, 78]. In addition, the beneficial effects of ALA were observed when LA:ALA ratio was close to 1:1, whereas the current $\omega 6$:$\omega 3$ ratio in the westernized diets is close to 16:1 [79].

Conclusion

Epidemiological studies and clinical trials indicate that there may be a beneficial effect of ALA on the primary and secondary prevention of CAD.

A 4:1 ratio in a dietary pattern consistent with a modified diet of Crete has also been shown to decrease total mortality and re-infarction rates. A ratio of 1:1 or less of LA:ALA suppresses IL-1β, IL-6, TNF-α, and CRP. CRP is a potent inflammatory factor that increases the risk of CAD. However, in order to decrease the ratio of LA:ALA in current Western diets, it would be necessary to decrease LA intake and increase ALA by changing the cooking oils or produce foods fortified with ALA.

References

1   Thies F, Garry JMC, Yaqoob P, Rerkasem K, Williams J, Shearman CP, Gallagher PJ, Calder PC, Grimble RF: Association of n-3 polyunsaturated fatty acids with stability of atherosclerotic plaques: A randomised controlled trial. Lancet 2003;361:477–485.
2   Kris-Etherton PM, Harris WS, Appel LJ: Fish consumption, fish oil, omega-3 fatty acids and cardiovascular disease. Arterioscler Thromb Vasc Biol 2003;23:e20–e30.
3   Nestel PJ: Fish oil and cardiovascular disease: Lipids and arterial function. Am J Clin Nutr 2000; 71:228–231.
4   Harper CR, Jacobson TA: The fats of life. The role of omega-3 fatty acids in the prevention of coronary heart disease. Arch Intern Med 2001;161:2185–2192.
5   Department of the Environment, Food and Rural Affairs: The National Food Survey. London, HM Stationary Office, 2001.
6   Kris-Etherton PM, Taylor DS, Yu-Poth S, Huth P, Moriarty K, Fishell V, Hargrove RL, Zhao G, Etherton TD: Polyunsaturated fatty acids in the food chain in the United States. Am J Clin Nutr 2000;71(suppl 1):179S–188S.
7   USDA Nutrient data laboratory. Available at: http://www.nalusda.gov/fnic/foodcomp.
8   Brenna JT: Efficiency of conversion of α-linolenic acid to long chain n-3 fatty acids in man. Curr Opin Clin Nutr Metab Care 2002;5:127–132.
9   Emken EA, Adlot RO, Gulley RM: Dietary linoleic acid influences desaturation and acylation of deuterium-labeled linoleic and linolenic acids in young adult males. Biochim Biophys Acta 1994; 1213:277–288.
10 Simopoulos AP: Omega-3 fatty acids in health and disease and in growth and development. Am J Clin Nutr 1991;54:438–463.
11 Simopoulos AP: Essential fatty acids in health and disease. Am J Clin Nutr 1999;70(suppl): 560S–569S.
12 Ross R: Atherosclerosis – An inflammatory disease. N Engl J Med 1999;340:115–126.
13 Libby P: Current concepts of the pathogenesis of the acute coronary syndromes. Circulation 2001; 104:365–372.
14 Ridker PM: On evolutionary biology, inflammation, infection, and the causes of atherosclerosis. Circulation 2002;105:2–4.
15 Pearson TA, Mensah GA, Alexander RW, Anderson JL, Cannon RO, Criqui M, Fadl YY, Fortmann SP, Hong Y, Myers GL, Rifai N, Smith S Jr, Taubert K, Tracy RP, Vinicor F: Markers of inflammation and cardiovascular disease: application to clinical and public health practice: A statement for health care professionals from the Centers for Disease Control and Prevention and the American Heart Association. Circulation 2003;107:499–511.
16 Lagrand WK, Viser CA, Hermens WT, Niessen HW, Verheugt FW, Wolbink GJ, Hack CE: C-reactive protein as a cardiovascular risk factor: More than an epiphenomenon? Circulation 1999;100:96–102.
17 Danesh J, Whincu P, Walker M, Lennon L, Thomson A, Appleby P, Gallimore JR, Pepys MB: Low grade inflammation and coronary heart disease: Prospective study and updated meta-analyses. BMJ 2000;321:199–204.

18 Tracy RP: Inflammation in cardiovascular disease: Cart, horse, or both? Circulation 1998;97: 2000–2002.

19 Castell JV, Gomez-Lechon MJ, David M, Andus T, Geiger T, Trullenque R, Fabra R, Heinrich PC: Interleukin-6 is the major regulator of acute phase protein synthesis in adult human hepatocytes. FEBS Lett 1989;242:237–239.

20 Mohamed-Ali V, Goodrick S, Rawesh A, Katz DR, Miles JM, Yudkin JS, Klein S, Coppack SW: Subcutaneous adipose tissue releases interleukin-6, but not tumor necrosis factor-alpha, in vivo. J Clin Endocrinol Metab 1997;82:4196–4200.

21 Yudkin JS, Stehouwer CD, Emeis JJ, Coppack SW: C-reactive protein in healthy subjects: associations with obesity, insulin resistance and endothelial dysfunction: A potential role of cytokines originating from adipose tissue? Arterioscler Thromb Vasc Biol 1999;19:972–978.

22 Simopoulos AP: Omega-3 fatty acids in inflammation and autoimmune diseases. J Am Coll Nutr 2002;21:495–505.

23 Guallar E, Aro A, Jimenez FJ, Martin-Moreno JM, Salminen I, Van't VP, Kardinaal AF, Gomez-Aracena J, Martin BC, Kohlmeier L, Kark JD, Mazaev VP, Ringstad J, Guillen J, Riemersma RA, Huttunen JK, Tham M, Kok FJ: Omega-3 fatty acids in adipose tissue and risk of myocardial infarction: The EURAMIC Study. Arterioscler Thromb Vasc Biol 1999;19:1111–1118.

24 Djousse L, Pankow JS, Eckfeldt JH, Folsom AR, Hopkins PH, Province MA, Hong Y, Ellison CR: Relation between dietary linolenic acid and coronary artery disease in the National Heart, Lung, and Blood Institute Family Heart Study. Am J Clin Nutr 2001;74:612–619.

25 Hu FB, Stampfer MJ, Mason JE, Stampfer MJ, Manson JE, Rimm EB, Wolk A, Colditz GA, Hennekens CH, Willett WC: Dietary intake of alpha-linolenic acid and risk of fatal ischemic heart disease among women. Am J Clin Nutr 1999;69:890–897.

26 Ascherio A, Rimm EB, Ciovannucci EL, Spiegelman D, Stamfer M, Willett WC: Dietary fat and risk of coronary heart disease in men: Cohort follow up study in the United States. BMJ 1996; 313:84–90.

27 Oomen CM, Ocke MC, Feskens EJM, Kok FJ, Kromhout D: α-linolenic acid intake is not beneficially associated with 10-y risk of coronary artery disease incidence: the Zutphen Elderly Study. Am J Clin Nutr 2001;74:457–463.

28 De Longeril M, Salen P, Martin JL, Monjaud I, Delaye J, Mamelle N: Mediterranean diet, traditional risk factors, and the rate of cardiovascular complications after myocardial infarction. Final report of the Lyon Diet heart Study. Circulation 1999;99:779–785.

29 Singh RB, Dubnov G, Niaz MA, Ghosh S, Singh R, Rastogi SS, Manor O, Pella D, Berry EM: Effect of an Indo-Mediterranean diet on progression of coronary artery disease in high risk patients (Indo-Mediterranean Diet Heart Study): A randomised single-blind trial. Lancet 2002; 360:1455–1461.

30 Singh RB, Niaz MA, Sharma JP, Kumar R, Rastogi V, Moshiri M: Randomized, double blind, placebo-controlled trial of fish oil and mustard oil in patients with suspected acute myocardial infarction: the Indian experiment of infarct survival. Cardiovasc Drugs Ther 1997;11:485–491.

31 Bebelmans WJE, Broer J, Feskens EJM, Smit AJ, Muskiet FAJ, Lefrandt JD, Bom VJJ, May JF, de Jong BM: Effect of an increased intake of α-linolenic acid and group nutritional education on cardiovascular risk factors: The Mediterranean Alpha-Linolenic Enriched Groningen Dietary Intervention (MARGARIN) study. Am J Clin Nutr 2002;75:221–227.

32 Allman-Farinelli MA, Hall D, Kingham K, Pang D, Petocz P, Favaloro EJ: Comparison of the effects of two low fat diets with different α-linolenic:linoleic acid ratios on coagulation and fibrinolysis. Atherosclerosis 1999;142:159–168.

33 Li D, Sinclair A, Wilson A, Nakkote S, Kelly F, Abedin L, Mann N, Turner A: Effect of dietary α-linolenic acid on thrombotic risk factors in vegetarian men. Am J Clin Nutr 1999;69:872–882.

34 Archer SL, Green D, Chamberlain M, Dyer AR, Liu K: Association of dietary fish and n-3 fatty acid intake with hemostatic factors in the Coronary Artery Risk Development in Young Adults (CARDIA) Study. Arterioscler Thromb Vasc Biol 1998;18:1118–1123.

35 Mutanen M, Freese R: Fats, lipids and blood coagulation. Curr Opin Lipidol 2001;12:25–29.

36 Renaud S, Morazain R, Godsey F, Dumont E, Thevenon C, Martin JL, Mendy F: Nutrients, platelet function and composition in nine groups of French and British farmers. Atherosclerosis 1986;60:37–48.

37 Pang D, Allman-Farinelli MA, Wong T, Barnes R, Kingham KM: Replacement of linoleic acid with alpha-linolenic acid does not alter blood lipids in normolipidaemic men. Br J Nutr 1998; 80:163–167.

38 Sanderson P, Finnegan YE, Williams CM, Calder PC, Burdge G, Wootton SA, Griffin BA, Millward J, Pegge NC, Bemelmans WJE: UK Food Standards Agency α-linolenic acid workshop report. Br J Nutr 2002;88:573–579.

39 Roper RL, Phipps RP: Prostaglandin E2 regulation of the immune response. Adv Prost Thromb Leuk Res 1994;22:101–111.

40 Harris WS: n-3 fatty acids and serum lipoproteins: Human studies. Am J Clin Nutr 1997; (suppl 5):1645S–1654S.

41 Roper RL, Brown DM, Phipps RP: Prostaglandin E2 promotes B lymphocyte Ig isotype switching to IgE. J Immunol 1995;154:162–170.

42 Tsang WM, Weyman C, Smith AD: Effect of fatty acid mixtures on phytohaem-agglutinin-stimulated lymphocytes of different species. Biochem Soc Trans 1977;5:153–154.

43 Offner H, Clausen J: Inhibition of lymphocyte response to stimulants induced by unsaturated fatty acids and prostaglandins in multiple sclerosis. Lancet 1974;2:1204–1205.

44 Mertin J, Hughes D: Specific inhibitory action of polyunsaturated fatty acids on lymphocyte transformation induced by PHA and PPD. Int Arch Allergy Appl Immunol 1975;48:203–210.

45 Weyman C, Belin J, Smith AD, Thompson RHS: Linoleic acid as an immunosuppressive agent. Lancet 1975;ii:33.

46 Calder PC, Bond JA, Bevan SJ, Hunt SV, Newsholme EA: Effect of fatty acids on the proliferation of concanavalin A-stimulated rat lymph node lymphocytes. Int J Biochem 1991;23: 579–588.

47 Calder PC, Newsholme EA: Unsaturated fatty acids suppress interleukin-2 production and transferrin receptor expression by concanavalin A-stimulated rat lymphocytes. Mediat Inflamm 1992;1:107–115.

48 Brouard C, Pascaud M: Modulation of rat and human lymphocyte function by n-6 and n-3 polyunsaturated fatty acids and acetylsalicylic acid. Ann Nutr Metab 1993;37:146–159.

49 Santoli D, Phillips PD, Colt TL, Zurier RB: Suppression of interleukin-2-dependent human T cell growth in vitro by prostaglandin E (PGE) and their precursor fatty acids. J Clin Invest 1990;85: 424–432.

50 Calder PC, Newsholme EA: Polyunsaturated fatty acids suppress human peripheral blood lymphocyte proliferation and interleukin-2 production. Clin Sci 1992;82:695–700.

51 Soyland E, Nenseter MS, Braathen L, Drevon CA: Very long chain n-3 and n-6 polyunsaturated fatty acids inhibit proliferation of human T lymphocytes in vitro. Eur J Clin Invest 1993;23: 112–121.

52 Purasiri P, McKechnie A, Heys SD, Eremin O: Modulation in vitro of human natural cytotoxicity, lymphocyte proliferative response to mitogens and cytokine production by essential fatty acids. Immunology 1997;92:166–172.

53 Khalfoun B, Thibault G, Lacord M, Gruel Y, Bardos P, Lebranchu Y: Docosahexaenoic and eicosapentaenoic acids inhibit human lymphoproliferative responses in vitro but not the expression of T cell surface activation markers. Scand J Immunol 1996;43:248–256.

54 Watanabe S, Hayashi H, Onozaki K, Okuyama H: Effect of dietary γ-linolenate/linoleate balance on lipopolysaccharide-induced tumor necrosis factor production in mouse macrophages. Life Sci 1991;48:2013–2020.

55 Turek JJ, Schoenlein IA, Bottoms GD: The effect of dietary n-3 and n-6 fatty acids on tumor necrosis factor-α production and leucine aminopeptidase levels in rat peritoneal macrophages. Prostaglandins Leukot Essent Fatty Acids 1991;43:141–149.

56 Hubbard NE, Chapkin RS, Erickson KL: Effect of dietary linseed oil on tumoricidal activity and eicosanoid production in murine macrophages. Lipids 1994;29:651–655.

57 Marshall LA, Johnston PV: The influence of dietary essential fatty acids on rat immunocompetent cell prostaglandin synthesis and mitogen-induced blastogenesis. J Nutr 1985;115:1572–1580.

58 Jeffery NM, Sanderson P, Sherrington EJ, Newsholme EA, Calder PC: The ratio of n-6 to n-3 polyunsaturated fatty acids in the rat diet alters serum lipid levels and lymphocyte functions. Lipids 1996;31:737–745.

59   Kelley DS, Branch LB, Love JE, Taylor PC, Rivera YM, Iacono JM: Dietary α-linolenic acid and immunocompetence in humans. Am J Clin Nutr 1991;53:40–46.

60   Caughey GE, Mantzioris E, Gibson RA, Cleland LG, James MJ: The effect on human tumor necrosis factor-α and interleukin-1β production of diets enriched in n-3 fatty acids from vegetable oil or fish oil. Am J Clin Nutr 1996;63:116–122.

61   Chan JK, McDonald BE, Gerrard JM, Bruce VB, Weaver BJ, Holub BJ: Effect of dietary r-linolenic acid and its ratio to linoleic acid on platelet and plasma fatty acids and thrombogenesis. Lipids 1993;28:811–817.

62   Thies F, Nebe-von-Caron G, Powell JR, Yaqoob P, Newsholme EA, Calder PC: Dietary supplementation with γ-linolenic acid or fish oil decreases T lymphocyte proliferation in healthy older humans. J Nutr 2001;131:1918–1927.

63   Thies F, Nebe-von-Caron G, Powell JR, Yaqoob P, Newsholme EA, Calder PC: Dietary supplementation with eicosapentaenoic acid, but not with other long-chain n-3 or n-6 polyunsaturated fatty acids, decreases natural killer cell activity in healthy subjects aged >55 y. Am J Clin Nutr 2001;73:539–548.

64   Rallidis LS, Paschos G, Liakos GK, Velissaridou AH, Anastasiadis G, Zampelas A: Dietary α-linolenic acid decreases C-reactive protein, serum amyloid A and interleukin-6 in dyslipidaemic patients. Atherosclerosis, in press.

65   Hutchinson IV, Pravica V, Hajeer A, Sinnott PJ: Identification of high and low responders to allographs. Rev Immunogent 1999;1:323–333.

66   Grimble RF: Nutritional modulation of immune function. Proc Nutr Soc 2001;60:389–397.

67   Fishman D, Faulds G, Jeffery R, Mohamed-Ali V, Yudkin JS, Humphries S, Woo P: The effect of novel polymorphisms in the interleukin-6 (IL-6) gene on IL-6 transcription and plasma IL-6 levels, and an association with systemic-onset juvenile chronic arthritis. J Clin Invest 1998;102:1369–1376.

68   Wilson AG, di Giovine F, Duff GW: Genetics of tumor necrosis factor-W in autoimmune, infectious and neoplastic disease. J Inflamm 1995;45:1–12.

69   McGuire W, Hill AV, Allsopp CE, Greenwood BM, Kwaitskowski D: Variations in the TNF-M promoter region associated with susceptibility to cerebral maralia. Nature 1994;371:508–511.

70   Stuber F, Petersen M, Bokelmann FA: Genomic polymorphisms within the tumor necrosis factor locus influences plasma TNF-p concentrations and outcomes of patients with sepsis. Crit Care Med 1996:24; 381–384.

71   Majetschak M, Flohe S, Obertavke V, Scroder J, Staubach K, Nast-Kolb D, Schade V, Stuber F: Relationships of a TNF gene polymorphism to severe sepsis in trauma patients. Ann Surg 1999;230:207–214.

72   Grimble RF, Howell WM, O'Reilly G, Turner SJ, Markovic O, Hirrell S, East JM, Calder PC: The ability of fish oil to suppress tumor necrosis factor alpha production by peripheral blood mononuclear cells in healthy men is associated with polymorphisms in genes that influence tumor necrosis factor alpha production. Am J Clin Nutr 2002;76:454–459.

73   Curtiss LK, Boisvert WA: Apolipoprotein E and atherosclerosis. Curr Opin Lipidol 2000;11:243–251.

74   Delomenie C, Wautier-Pepin MP, Chappey O, Wautier JL: Modulation of human endothelial cell activation by antiproliferative cytokines: Exploration of arachidonic acid and intracellular cytokine pathways as possible mechanisms of action. Exp Cell Res. 1993;207:122–130.

75   Ohhashi K, Takahashi T, Watanabe S, Kobayashi T, Okuyama H, Hata N, Misawa Y: Effect of replacing a high linoleate oil with a low linoleate, high alpha-linolenate oil, as compared with supplementing EPA or DHA, on reducing lipid mediator production in rat polymorphonuclear leukocytes. Biol Pharm Bull 1998;21:558–564.

76   Caughey GE, Pouliot M, Cleland LG, James MJ: Regulation of tumor necrosis factor alpha and interleukin-1 beta synthesis by thromboxane A2 in non-adherent human monocytes. J Immunol 1997;158:351–358.

77   Valsta LM, Salminen I, Aro A, Mutanen M: Alpha-linolenic acid in rapeseed oil partly compensates for the effect of fish restriction on plasma chain n-3 fatty acids. Eur J Clin Nutr 1996;50:229–235.

78   Burdge GC, Jones AE, Wootton SA: Eicosapentaenoic and docosapenaenoic acids are the principal products of α-linolenic acid metabolism in young men. Br J Nutr 2002;88:355–363.
79   Simopoulos AP: The importance of the ratio of omega-6/omega-3 essential fatty acids. Biomed Pharmacother 2002;56:365–379.

Antonis Zampelas, PhD
Laboratory of Nutrition and Clinical Dietetics
Department of Nutrition and Dietetics, Harokopio University
El. Venizelou 70, GR–17671 Athens (Greece)
Tel. +30 210 9549 153, Fax +30 210 9549 141, E-Mail azampelas@hua.gr

Simopoulos AP, Cleland LG (eds): Omega–6/Omega–3 Essential Fatty Acid Ratio:
The Scientific Evidence. World Rev Nutr Diet. Basel, Karger, 2003, vol 92, pp 109–132

....

The Japan Society for Lipid Nutrition Recommends to Reduce the Intake of Linoleic Acid

A Review and Critique of the Scientific Evidence

Tomohito Hamazaki[a], *Harumi Okuyama*[b]

[a] Department of Clinical Application, Institute of Natural Medicine,
  Toyama Medical and Pharmaceutical University, Sugitani, Toyama-shi, Toyama, and
[b] Department of Preventive Nutraceutical Sciences, Graduate School of Pharmaceutical
  Sciences, Nagoya City University, Nagoya, Japan

On September 6, 2002, the Japan Society for Lipid Nutrition (JSLN) adopted a proposal that nutritional recommendations should be changed to a new direction so as to reduce the intake of linoleic acid (LA) for the prevention of coronary heart disease (CHD) and other chronic diseases, but recognized that evidence from clinical studies is not enough to set an adequate daily intake of LA in terms of energy % (en%) (table 1). In this chapter, we explain why LA should be reduced, based mainly on reviewing clinical studies. We would like to remind non-Japanese readers that the recommended daily intake of LA discussed below might be applicable only for those whose intake of omega–3 fatty acids is comparable to those of average Japanese (2.6 g/day as a total including about 1 g of EPA plus DHA [1]). This level is probably enough for preventive purposes, and we did not argue for further increasing omega–3 fatty acid intake in healthy subjects.

The Selling Points of Linoleic Acid

Since about 40 years ago, nutritionists have recommended increasing the polyunsaturated/saturated (P/S) ratio of ingested fatty acids, and edible-oil-producing companies in Japan have been advertising LA as healthy. The consumption of LA has increased roughly threefold (fig. 1) during this period.

Table 1. Recommendation by the Japan Society for Lipid Nutrition (JSLN) to reduce linoleic acid intake and to improve the ingredient labeling of lipid-rich foods (September, 2002) [2]

1	JSLN recommends to reduce the intake of linoleic acid
	The essential amount is more or less 1 en%, and reducing the linoleic acid intake from the current levels in the industrialized countries (>5–7 en%) is recommended
2	JSLN recommends to lower the linoleic acid levels in infant formulae to the levels of mother's milk
	The recent LA content in mother's milk is as follows: 13% of the total fatty acids in Japan, 9% in Germany, and 8% in Australia and Sweden
3	JSLN recommends to label individual species names for edible oils (e.g. soybean oil, high-oleic safflower oil, hydrogenated soybean oil, etc.) instead of collective names (such as plant oil, animal oil and processed oil)
4	JSLN recommends to label the content of omega–3 and omega–6 fatty acids for foods containing more than 50% (w/w) lipids

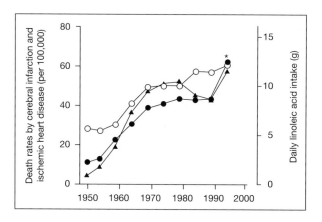

Fig. 1. Changes over time in LA intake and the death rates from ischemic heart disease and cerebral infarction in Japan. Data were adopted from references [1] and [3]. *: The death rates of ischemic heart disease and cerebral infarction apparently increased in 1995 because of the revision of death certificate rules in 1995. Open circle = Daily LA intake; closed triangle = cerebral infarction; closed circle = ischemic heart disease.

In these several years, such advertisements have disappeared, but the majority of people still believe that high-LA plant oils are better for their health than animal fat. There were (or maybe still 'are') two selling points for LA during those years of its active advertisement. One is its essentiality, and the other is its ability to lower blood cholesterol.

Its deficiency impairs skin integrity, growth and reproduction. More or less 1 en% of LA is necessary. However, the average Japanese intake of LA is around 6 en%. Besides, there have never been LA-deficient patients reported in Japan except for those who were under total parenteral nutrition, which was reported a few decades ago. The same also holds true in the Western world [4]. A completely fat-free diet changed the fatty acid composition of their blood samples of volunteers, increasing the concentration of eicosatrienoic acid omega-9, but they developed no LA deficiency symptoms at all [5]. Actually, people have a large stock of LA in their body. On the average, people have 20 kg of fat or more, of which 15% is LA. Taken together, the first selling point is practically meaningless. People have too much LA.

High blood cholesterol levels is a well-known risk factor for CHD, but, if the total death rates are taken into account, high cholesterol levels may not be a sizable risk factor in Japan. It is not as simple as 'the lower the cholesterol levels, the better', at least in Japan where the death rate from CHD is one quarter that of the United States and one eighth that of Western European countries. Recently, the relationship between total cholesterol levels and total death rates became available from epidemiological studies with 10,000 general citizens or more in Japan. According to the data of Osaka Prefecture [6] the cholesterol levels of 240–280 mg/dl (6.2–7.3 mmol/l) were the best in terms of the total death rate when both males and females are combined (fig. 2a). A research study on residents from all over Japan [7] revealed that the cholesterol levels of 240–260 mg/dl (6.2–6.7 mmol/l) were the best (fig. 2b). The relationship between the blood cholesterol and total death rate in Hukui citizens was more striking [8]. Although the deaths from cancer during the first few years after blood sampling were not excluded, there was no significant correlation between the cholesterol levels and the total death rates in women, but in men the higher the cholesterol levels, the lower the total death rates (fig. 2c). These results suggest that there is no need to lower the total cholesterol levels up to 260–280 mg/dl (6.7–7.3 mmol/l) in Japanese people, because those with the highest blood cholesterol (>250 mg/dl, 6.5 mmol/l) lived the longest of all. Here again, LA lost its selling point. It is also known that too much LA intake decreased HDL-cholesterol levels [9, 10].

Metabolites of Linoleic Acid – What Kinds of Drugs Are Doctors Prescribing Everyday?

LA is converted to arachidonic acid (AA) through two cycles of desaturation and one cycle of chain elongation, and these are integrated into cell membranes in various tissues. Where cells are stimulated by one way or another, phospholipase A_2 becomes available and releases AA from membrane phospholipids. Free AA is then converted into eicosanoids such as prostaglandins (PG), leukotrienes (LT), thromboxanes (TX), etc. (fig. 3). Certain amounts of

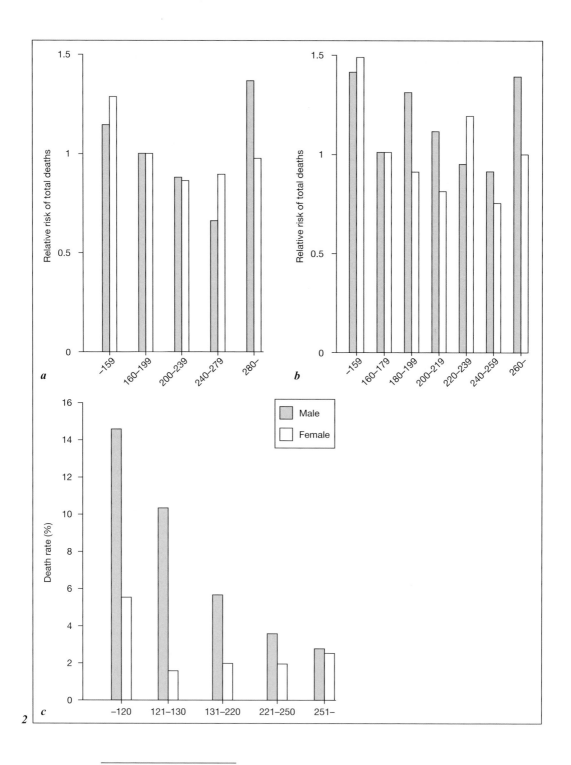

eicosanoids are necessary for sustaining life, but if eicosanoids are overproduced, they cause a wide variety of pathological conditions. When a patient has fever, pain or inflammation in general, the doctor very often prescribes a nonsteroidal anti-inflammatory drug (NSAID), e.g. aspirin, the most famous NSAID for the treatment of heart attack and sometimes for prevention of even colon cancer [11]. There is no panacea in the world, but probably steroidal anti-inflammatory drugs (SAID) may be considered to be near panacea because they can change pathological conditions from inflammation, to allergy, to cancer. SAIDs exert their effects, at least in part, by preventing AA release and eicosanoid formation. Almost all doctors prescribe NSAIDs and/or SAIDs every day. But, is reducing LA intake and lowering AA levels in cell membranes a much more effective and safer method to ameliorate AA cascade-related pathological conditions than using NSAIDs and SAIDs? NSAIDs and SAIDs can indeed act very fast compared with LA reduction; however, the effects of those drugs do not last long, and once people stop using those drugs their conditions reverse to the previous pathological state immediately [12].

In this volume, there are many chapters describing the beneficial effects of omega–3 fatty acids. There are quite a few mechanisms of action of omega–3 fatty acids, but the competition between the omega–6 and omega–3 fatty acids at steps of elongation, desaturation, esterification into phospholipids, their release, conversion to eicosanoids (lipid mediators) and at their receptors is the major theme that explains why omega–3 fatty acids are necessary for the prevention of CHD and other chronic diseases [12]. Accepting the usefulness of omega–3 fatty acids is nearly equal to admitting the risk of excessive LA intake. Until several decades ago, LA and its derivatives, omega–6 eicosanoids, had been useful, but now they are not so any more.

From here on, we analyze the results of large-scale epidemiological studies on LA intake and CHD, which are mostly from Western countries. However, one important concern about those studies needs to be addressed before going into detail.

Fig. 2. Relationship between the total serum cholesterol levels and total death rates. The x-axis indicates serum cholesterol levels of study subjects. *a* Residents of Osaka-prefecture (9,662 males and females at 40–79 years of age) were followed up for 10.7 years on average, and the total death rates were calculated. Deaths were not counted in for the first 2 years [6]. *b* 9,726 males and females over 30 years of age, collected from 300 districts all over Japan, were followed up for 14 years. Deaths were not counted in for the first 5 years [7]. *c* 26,249 residents of Hukui city were followed up for 5 years. All deaths were counted from the first year [8]. There is a possibility that those people who had already cancer at blood sample collection and died during the study period might have lower serum cholesterol levels because of their cancer. In all cases (*a*), (*b*) and (*c*), there were more cancer deaths in the lowest cholesterol levels and more CHD deaths in the highest cholesterol levels.

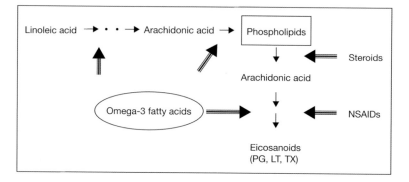

Fig. 3. Eicosanoid production and its inhibition. Arrows indicate the site of inhibitory effects. Eicosanoids are involved in a wide range of pathological conditions if produced in excess. NSAIDs and steroid hormones can quickly change the pathological conditions and/or reduce symptoms induced by eicosanoid formation even when the tissue AA levels are high. However, the effects of these drugs are not long-lasting. In this sense, reduction of the AA levels (or enhancement of natural inhibitors (omega–3 fatty acids)) by dietary manipulation induces essential changes in tissue pathology [12].

Were α-Linolenic Acid Intakes Adequate for the Subjects in Western Epidemiological Studies?

In discussing the effects of LA intake on various endpoints, there seems to be a serious problem in the Western epidemiological studies; namely, the existence of a significant part of the population whose α-linolenic acid (ALA) intakes were below the essential level. We estimated the daily intake of ALA from several epidemiological studies [13–18], some of which are cited in tables 2 and 3 (see the next two sections for their details). To our surprise, study subjects of those reports ingested only 0.3–0.5 en% of ALA on average. (Just for reference, Japanese people eat 1.2 en% on average [1].) The daily required amounts of ALA were calculated to be 0.2–0.3 en%, which was an estimate for treating 9 patients under omega–3 fatty acid-deficiency after a long period of parenteral nutrition containing almost no omega–3 fatty acids [19]. These estimated values are very close to daily intakes of study subjects [13–18]. This means that a significant proportion of the study subjects were close to omega–3 fatty acid deficiency, since average Western people do not eat fish so frequently.

It has been reported that the rate of sudden death is about twice as high in the subjects of the lowest quartile of total omega–3 long-chain fatty acids in whole blood lipids than those of the second lowest quartile [32]; the second lowest quartile probably corresponds to those who eat fish once a week or less. Furthermore, the risk of ischemic stroke increased nearly twice in the group whose fish intake was less than once a month compared with 1–3 times a month [33]. The fact that such small increases in the intake of omega–3 long-chain fatty acids induce a drastic change in cardiocerebrovascular disease incidence also suggests that omega–3 fatty acid deficiency should be regarded as a real threat to Western people. In contrast, LA intake is quite enough compared with the necessary amount (1 en%) even in the group with the lowest intake of LA (tables 2, 3).

We can easily increase LA intake by increasing plant oil consumption. Old type safflower oil contained almost 80% LA with essentially no ALA, but soybean oil has more than 50% LA and also 7–8% ALA. Consequently, the method of enhancing LA intake sometimes increases ALA intake at the same time. This point is important because LA increase may be good only through preventing omega–3 fatty acid deficiency, as discussed below.

Coronary Heart Disease and LA – Epidemiological Studies

Cohort and case-control studies describing the relationship between LA intake and CHD are listed in table 2. The papers that regard LA as a positive and negative risk factor are marked with '+' and '−', respectively, in the table. The numbers of '+' and '−' are similar, so it is difficult to decide whether LA is good for the heart or bad. However, a close look at the table reveals a few common characteristics in the '−' papers; they are generally old and had all been published before 1993; subjects were all males and younger than 65 years of age (partly because the life span was shorter when studies were performed). These points are in good contrast to the '+' papers. The situation is similar in the intervention trials shown in table 3.

It seems rather difficult to reconcile these '+' and '−' papers, but perhaps the best way is to assume a J curve effect of LA on CHD. Pedersen et al. [25] showed there was a J curve effect of LA content in the adipose tissue on the odds ratio of first myocardial infarction. They calculated that the second lowest quintile of the adipose LA content (9.4–10.5%, estimated to be around 4.4–5.2 en%; see the estimation method shown in the legend to table 2) had the lowest odds ratio (odds ratios of low to high quintiles were 1.0, 0.57, 0.90, 1.39 and 2.13, and p for trend was <0.02). According to a recent paper by Djoussé et al. [13], LA intake of the middle tertile, 6.65 g/day (about 3 en%), had the lowest incidence of CHD after adjusting many confounding factors including ALA (α- and γ-linolenic acids were not differentiated, but γ-linolenic acid must be negligible in foods) (tables 2, 4). It is, therefore, conceivable that 3–4 en% may be the best range of LA for the heart. We could also reach a similar conclusion from the intervention studies shown in the next section.

Table 2. Linoleic acid (LA) and coronary heart disease (epidemiological studies)

First author country where investigation was done	Reference	Publication year	Years of investigation (period of investigation)	End points	n cases (n controls) (total participants)	Age	Measured fraction of PUFA	LA en% of the control group* (LA% of adipose tissue)	Is LA a positive risk factor?	Notes
Case control study										
Miettinen, Finland	20	1982	5–7 years	AMI	33 (64) (M)	40–55 y	serum lipids (prospective)	n.a.	–	LA% in the serum PL were lower in the AMI group than in the control group (23.04 vs. 26.15%)
Válek, Czechoslovakia	21	1985	–	AMI acute phase	80 survivors, 23 deaths within 3 months 23 controls (M)	below 65 (average: 53)	serum total lipids 4–7 days after admission	n.a.	–	LA% in serum of those who died between 2 weeks and 3 months were lower than the controls or survivors
Wood, UK	22	1987	1983–1984	first angina and AMI	125AP + 85AMI (430) (M)	35–54	adipose tissue, platelet membranes collected in hospital for AMI	LA% of the low Q5 of the adipose tissue was below 7.8% (3.2 en% (E))	–	the risk of angina pectoris was 3.2 times higher in the low Q5 of adipose tissue LA than in the high
Roberts, UK	23	1993	–	sudden deaths	84 (292) (M)	25–64	adipose tissue	LA% of the low Q5 of the adipose tissue was below 9.5% (4.5 en% (E))	–	the risk of sudden death was 4.4 times higher in the low Q5 of adipose tissue LA than in the high
Hodgson, Australia	24	1993	10 months	CHD angiography	226 (M + F)	16–80 (average: 59)	adipose tissue and platelets	M: 6.8 en%; F: 7.6 en% (E) (M: 12.6%; F: 13.7%)	+	the LA concentration in the adipose tissue and platelets correlated with atherosclerosis
Pedersen, Norway	25	2000	1996 only	first AMI	100 (98) M + F (menopause)	45–75	adipose tissue	LA% of the low Q5 of the adipose tissue was below 9.4% (4.4 en% (E))	+ J curve	the risk of first AMI was 2.13 times higher in the high Q5 of adipose tissue LA than in the low; the risk of the second low Q5 (LA: 9.4–10.5%) is 0.57

Yli-Jama, Norway	26	2002	1995–1997	first AMI	103 (104) M+F (menopause)	45–75	serum free FA	n.a.	+	serum free LA concentration was higher in the patient group than in the control group
Cohort study										
Riemersma, UK	27	1986	1982–1983	death rates from CHD	Healthy subjects in 4 European a (total: 290 M)	40–49	adipose tissue	LA% of the high CHD death rates was 7.36–8.10% (2.9–3.5 en% (E))	–	inverse correlation between death rates and adipose tissue LA concentration
Blankenhorn, USA	28	1990	2 years	coronary angiography	control M pt in CLAS** 18 of 82 deteriorated	40–59	food questionnaire	baseline: 5.2–5.7 en% (E), deteriorated: 9.3 en%, not changed: 7.3 en%	+	the risk in the high LA T3 of deterioration of coronary arteries was 3.25 of the low T3
Tavendale, UK	29	1992	1984–1986	CHD deaths	(4,114) M+F	40–59	adipose tissue	average: M: 4.0 en%; F: 4.4 (E) (ad tissue LA%: M, 8.88; F, 9.37)	–	inverse correlation between mean adipose tissue LA% and CHD deaths in 22 areas in Scotland
Djoussé, USA	13	2001	1993–1995	CHD	(4,584) M+F	52 ± 14 45–69	food questionnaire	LA intakes of the low T3 were 3.86 g/d (1.4 en% (E))	J curve (see table 4)	the risks of CHD in the middle and high T3 were 0.60 and 0.61 of the low T3
Nakamura, Japan	30	2003	1994–1998	angina pectoris	residents of Kumihama area blood samples from 294	>39	total fatty acids of serum from healthy subjects	serum LA (mg/dL): 858 in a mercantile area, 823 in a farming, and 690 in a fishing	+ (see table 5)	in the fishing area (LA was low), the incidence of angina was 1/8 and 1/14 of the farming and mercantile areas, respectively

*LA intake was estimated from LA % in the adipose tissue using the formula shown below on the assumption that LA intake was 85% of the total PUFA intake and that LA % in the adipose tissue was the same as in the total fatty acid intake.

The estimation formula for LA intake: $Y = 1.85X - 6.35$, where Y is LA intake (% of the total fatty acids) and X is LA% in the adipose tissue. The equation was converted from figure 1 of reference [31].

**Cholesterol-Lowering Atherosclerosis Study.

AMI = Acute myocardial infarction; AP = angina pectoris; n.a. = not available; PL = phospholipids; Q5 = quintile; T3 = tertile.

Table 3. Intervention trials with changes in LA intake

First author, country where investigation was done	Study name	Reference	Publication year	Case no intervention/control	Age	Purpose	Intervention with regard to fatty acid	Period of intervention	LA intake (en%*) of the control group (LA% in the adipose tissue)	Is LA a positive risk factor?	Notes
Dayton, USA	–	34	1969	424/422 M	50–89	mostly primary prevention	P/S ↑	up to 8 years	(E) 5.5 en% (10.8%)	–	incidence of atherosclerotic disease including stroke was lower in the intervention group, but no difference in the total deaths
Leren, Norway	Oslo Diet-Heart Study	35	1970	206/206 M	30–64	secondary prevention	P/S ↑ cholesterol intake ↓	5 years with and next 6 years without intervention	55 g PUFA intake in the intervention group	–	5 years of intervention reduced AMI significantly; after 11 years AMI mortality was significantly reduced; no difference in the total death rates
Miettinen, Finland	Finnish Mental Hospital Study	36	1972	2,463/2,407 M + F	15 and over, including >75	primary prevention	P/S ↑	6 years	(E) 4.9 en% (9.8–10.2%)	–	AMI was significantly reduced only in men; no difference in the total death rates
Woodhill, Australia	Sydney Diet-Heart Study	37	1978	221/237 M	30–59	secondary prevention	P/S ↑	2–7 years	at the start (E) 5.6 en % during: 12.8 en% (intervention) and 7.6 en% (control)	+	overall survival was significantly better in the control group
Hjermann, Norway	Oslo Study	38	1981	604/628 M	40–49	primary prevention	saturated fat ↓, smoking ↓ PUFA slightly ↑	5 years	PUFA intakes in year 4 were 7.1 en% (control) and 8.3 en% (intervention)	0	risk of AMI and sudden deaths was 0.53; no difference in PUFA intake in the fourth year

Author	Study	Ref	Year	Subjects	Age	Prevention	Intervention	Duration	LA level	Effect	Outcome
Burr, UK	DART	39	1989	1,018/1,015 M	<70	secondary prevention	P/S ↑	2 years	plasma: 28.1% LA (intervention) 25.0% LA (control)	0	the number of total deaths was 111 in the intervention group (P/S = 0.78) and 113 in the control group (P/S = 0.4–0.44)
Frantz, USA	Minnesota Coronary Survey	40	1989	4,541/4516 M + F	no limits	primary prevention	5 en% PUFA (control) 15 en% PUFA (intervention)	up to 4.5 years average: 384 days	(E) 4.3 en% (control) 12.8 en% (intervention)	0	no difference in cardiovascular events and all-cause mortality
Strandberg, Finland	Helsinki Business men Study	41	1991	612/610 M	48 ± 4	primary prevention	P/S ↑ for 5 years, and no intervention for the next 10	5 years with and next 10 years without intervention	not available	+	risks of all-cause and cardiac deaths were 1.45 and 2.42, respectively, in the intervention group; see the text
de Lorgeril, France	Lyon Diet Heart Study	18	1998	302/303 M + F	<70	secondary prevention	LA intake 2/3, α-LNA intake 3 times	4 years	5.3 en% (control) 3.6 en% (intervention)	++	risks of all-cause and cardiac deaths were 0.44 and 0.35, respectively, in the low LA-high α-LNA group
Yoshiike, Japan	Follow-up Study of Controls for JLIT**	42	2001	4,918 M + F 10–20% were on diet therapy	35–70	primary prevention	P/S ↑	6 years	6 en% (average in Japan)	+	AMI increased 2.87 times in the group of subjects who received dietary education including high P/S

* Estimated from the equation shown in table 2.
**Originally this study was not an intervention trial, but it investigated the effects of dietary intervention.
(E) = Estimated values.

Table 4. Relations between LA/α-LNA intakes and CHD* [13]

Tertiles of LNA intakes	LA intakes, g/day		
	3.86 (1.09–5.23) 1.4 en%** n = 1,358	6.65 (5.24–8.24) 2.4 en% n = 1,567	11.66 (8.25–36.80) 4.2 en% n = 1,481
0.43 (0.13–0.56) 0.15 en% n = 1,445	1.0	0.69 (0.31–1.54)	–***
0.67 (0.57–0.78) 0.25 en% n = 1,338	0.91 (0.34–2.38)	0.83 (0.41–1.70)	1.04 (0.40–2.73)
1.07 (0.79–3.48) 0.39 en% n = 1,633	0.72 (0.02–28.96)	0.46 (0.17–1.21)	0.44 (0.17–1.17)

Determined by bootstrap logistic regression and adjusted for more than 20 risk factors.
*National Heart, Lung, and Blood Institute Family Heart Study.
**Estimated en% in case of 2,500 kcal/day (by the estimation method shown in table 2).
***Numbers in cells were too small for a stable estimate.

If we choose only the '–' papers from table 2, the LA intakes in the lowest LA or control groups were below 4 en%, which means the ideal LA intakes should be above 4 en%. However, this value (4 en%) must be overestimated because of the confounding factor of ALA deficiency as discussed in the previous section.

Very recently, Nakamura et al. [30] reported an interesting epidemiological study on three rural neighboring districts in Kyoto, Japan. The incidence of CHD and some important risk factors are shown in table 5. The incidence of angina pectoris in a fishing area was about one eighth of that of a farming area and about one 14th of a mercantile area, despite the fact that the smoking rate in the fishing area was higher than the other areas and that the total EPA content in serum was not significantly different among the areas (p = 0.07). The point is that LA and omega–6 fatty acids in serum were significantly lower in the fishing area than in the other areas. The authors of this study indicated that a lower intake of omega–6 PUFA and saturated fatty acids has a preventive effect on CHD [30].

Relationships between LA Intake and CHD (Intervention Studies)

Intervention studies have less confounding factors than epidemiological studies and can provide strong evidence. Here we summarize 10 intervention studies

Table 5. Population, CHD incidence and some risk factors of neighboring rural areas in Kyoto Prefecture [30]

	Mercantile area	Farming area	Fishing area	p value
Population and CHD incidence (/100,000 population/year)				
Population	2,069	7,571	2,944	
Positive stress ECG	290	238	34	<0.0001
Incidence of AMI	24	30	8	0.45
Incidence of angina pectoris	109	66	8	0.01
Clinical characteristics of the participants at annual checkups (mmol/l, mean ± SD)				
	(n = 95)	(n = 118)	(n = 81)	
Total cholesterol	5.62 ± 0.93	5.36 ± 0.88	5.13 ± 0.70*	0.0006
LDL-cholesterol	3.47 ± 0.85	3.21 ± 0.78	3.13 ± 0.60*	0.01
HDL-cholesterol	1.63 ± 0.36	1.66 ± 0.36	1.55 ± 0.34	0.08
Triglyceride	1.19 ± 0.57	1.13 ± 1.02	0.93 ± 0.46	0.07
Smoking rate, %	11.6	16.9	28.4	0.01
Serum fatty acid levels at annual checkups (mg/l, mean ± SD)				
Palmitic (16:0)	647 ± 146	658 ± 228	548 ± 116*#	<0.0001
Stearic (18:0)	217 ± 32	246 ± 66	198 ± 38*#	<0.0001
Oleic (18:1)	576 ± 137	570 ± 243	486 ± 118*#	0.002
LA (18:2ω–6)	858 ± 139	823 ± 202	690 ± 150*#	<0.0001
α-LNA(18:3ω–3)	22 ± 7	21 ± 9	17 ± 6*#	0.001
AA (20:4ω–6)	155 ± 26	142 ± 33	131 ± 28*#	<0.0001
EPA (20:5ω–3)	90 ± 40	84 ± 36	97 ± 46	0.07
DHA (22:6ω–3)	188 ± 50	175 ± 53	175 ± 61	0.14
ω–6/ω–3	3.44 ± 0.97	3.57 ± 1.30	3.07 ± 1.29*#	<0.0001

*,#Significantly different from the mercantile and farming areas, respectively.

after 1969 (table 3). The studies performed before 1969 were unable to show reduced CHD incidence by increasing LA intake. The last study in table 3 was originally an observational study [42], but some subjects of the study were treated with diet therapy, hence we included this in table 3. Studies reporting beneficial effects of high LA intake are all relatively old, included only males as subjects, and were unable to show reduced total death rate (table 3), which is in good contrast to those studies showing high LA intake as a positive risk factor for CHD [18, 37, 41, 42].

Intervention Studies Suggesting that LA Has Beneficial Effects in Decreasing the Risk for CHD

The typical example is the Finnish Mental Hospital Study (tables 3, 6) [36]. Two mental hospitals (N and K) took part in this study. For the first 6 years Hospital N raised the P/S ratio, and Hospital K served as a control. For the next 6 years, the two hospitals changed their roles. In order to increase the P/S ratio,

Table 6. Finnish Mental Hospital Study [36]

	Group	Number of patients[1]	All-cause deaths	CHD deaths	Cancer deaths	Cerebro-vascular deaths
Males						
	Intervention	902	188	34*	23	11
	Control	928	217	76	24	13
Females						
	Intervention	1,561	415	73**	51	33
	Control	1,479	465	129	38	35
Total[2]						
	Intervention	2,463	603	107	74	44
	Control	2,407	682	205	62	48

*$p < 0.002$; **$p < 0.1$ (age-adjusted in both cases).
[1]Total person-year divided by the study period of 6 years.
[2]Significance was not available.

whole milk was replaced with skim milk containing soybean oil; butter and hard margarine were replaced with soft margarine. The P/S ratio increased from 0.22–0.29 to 1.42–1.78. The LA content in the adipose tissue after 4–5 years was 26.9 and 10.2% in Hospitals N and K, and 9.8 and 32.0% 4–5 years after the cross-over in Hospitals N and K, respectively. Through raising the P/S ratio, deaths due to CHD were significantly reduced in males and tended to be reduced in females; total deaths were not reduced (table 6). The important point is that increasing soybean oil increased not only LA intake but also α-LNA intake. If PUFAs came mostly from soybean oil in the Finnish Mental Hospital Study, 2–3 g of ALA (0.7–1.1 en%) was estimated to be consumed in the experimental periods. Taking into account the background of possible ALA deficiency, this increase in ALA might be a hidden reason why CHD deaths were reduced. Extremely low intakes of LA might be as dangerous as too much LA, unless one eats fish.

Leren [35] randomized 412 men 1 to 2 years after a first acute myocardial infarction (AMI). For the experimental group he recommended to increase P/S ratios and reduce cholesterol intake. After 5 years, the total number of AMI had been reduced statistically significantly (61 vs. 81, $p = 0.05$). At the end of the study of 5 years, further dietary advice was discontinued, but after 11 years myocardial infarction mortality was found to be significantly reduced in the original diet group (32 vs. 57, $p = 0.004$) [35]. However, deaths from all causes were essentially equal between the two groups (101 in the experimental group

Table 7. Results during a 4-year follow-up of Lyon Hear Study [18]

	Control	Experimental	Risk ratio*	p value
Total deaths	24	14	0.44	0.03
Cardiac deaths	19	6	0.35	0.01
Cancer deaths	17	7	0.39	0.05
Cases diagnosed after 24 months	12	2		

*Adjusted for sex, age, smoking, blood cholesterol level, leukocyte count, and aspirin use at baseline.

vs. 108); this was due to an increase in unwitnessed deaths in the experimental group (14 vs. 7). Besides, the P/S ratio of the experimental group during the first 5 years was 2.4 (corresponding to 55 g of PUFA/day). This amount is too high to be of practical use.

According to the experiment performed by Dayton et al. [34], atherosclerosis-related events were significantly decreased (table 3). The LA in the adipose tissue was $10.9 \pm 3.5\%$ (estimated to be 5.5 en%) at baseline in the experimental group; that was increased to $33.6 \pm 5.5\%$ (about 15 en% or more?) in the subjects who rigidly adhered to the diet. Interestingly, in individuals on the experimental diet who died after prolonged experience in the study with high adherence to the diet, the AA concentration in atheroma phospholipids was significantly decreased (3.3 ± 1.4 vs. $7.1 \pm 0.7\%$ in the control group, $p < 0.05$) [34]. LA might compete with AA and reduce the tissue phospholipid levels of AA, but this phenomenon would be possible only with a tremendous amount of LA. Moreover, total deaths would not be reduced. LA and γ-linolenic acid as well as dihomo-γ-linolenic acid serve as precursors of AA in humans.

*Intervention Studies Suggesting that LA has Adverse
Effects in Decreasing the Risk for CHD*

The intervention study performed in France (Lyon Heart Study [18], see also chapter by de Lorgeril and Salen [this vol.]) used 605 AMI survivors below 70 years of age. One half of them were on a Mediterranean diet for the average period of 27 months. This experimental diet contained 3.6 en% LA and 0.81 en% of ALA, 68 and 300% of the control diet, respectively. The results were astonishing; although the blood cholesterol levels did not change in either group, the total death rate was reduced by 70% in the experimental group. This study was continued for 4 years as in the original protocol even after the disclosure of the results [43]. Table 7 summarizes the results at the end of this study. The risks of total death and cardiac death were reduced to 0.44 and 0.35, respectively, in the experimental group. Cancer incidence was also affected. For the first 2 years of the experiment, 5 cancer cases were found in each group, but there was a marked difference in the cancer incidence in favor of the experimental group for the last 2 years (table 7), although numbers of patients of both groups were rather small. It is likely that those subjects who had been in the last stage of preclinical cancer before the start of the study might have clinical signs and be diagnosed as cancer during the first 2 years. Consequently, the marked difference in cancer incidence in the last 2 years implies that the cancer-preventing effects (or the effects to delay the manifestation of clinical cancer) were brought about by reducing LA intake and/or increasing ALA intake.

The Lyon Heart Study was a successful one in terms of prevention of deaths and cardiac disease, but several factors were also intervened with in the experimental group, which makes it difficult to neglect the possibility that some other factors may be more important than changing the types of fatty acids ingested.

Contrary to the Lyon Heart Study, LA intakes were increased in the Helsinki Businessmen Study [41] (table 3). In a 5-year randomized, controlled trial with 1,222 healthy business executive men but with multiple cardiovascular risk factors, 612 entered to an intervention group. Nearly 70% of the intervention group took anti-hypertensive drugs and/or hypolipidemics as compared with only 15% in the control group. Subjects in the intervention group were intensively treated with dietetic and hygienic measures. The following dietary instructions were given: reduction of intakes of calories, saturated fat, cholesterol, alcohol and sugar, and increments in polyunsaturated fats (mainly as soft margarine), fish, chicken, veal and vegetables. At the end of the 5-year intervention, the coronary incidence tended to be higher in the intervention group than in the control group (3.1 vs. 1.5%), although total CHD risk was reduced by 46% in the intervention group as compared with the control group at the end of the trial [44]. During the post-trial 5 years, the risk factor and medication differences were largely leveled off between the groups [44]. During the 5-year trial and the 10-year post-trial period, the mortalities from CHD and all cause death were 2.4- and 1.4-fold higher in the intervention group than in the control group, respectively [41].

It is not quite clear yet why the death rates were increased in the intervention group. However, the investigators tried to increase a PUFA intake in the intervention group by recommending soft margarine [44]. Once taught that soft margarine containing a lot of LA is better for your health, lay people may have difficulty switching back to butter or hard margarine. It is likely that subjects in the intervention group still continued to take soft margarine even after the trial.

Because the subjects in the intervention group were recommended to eat more fish, there remains a possibility that mercury contamination in the lakes of Eastern Finland [45] might have something to do with an increased CHD incidence in the intervention trial, but this toxic effect of mercury might have been cancelled out by the beneficial effects of omega–3 PUFA contained in fish [46] or simply might not be related to CHD [47]. Consequently, it is very likely that the increased LA intake from soft margarine was the major cause for the increased death rate in the Helsinki Businessmen Study.

Statins are well-known blood cholesterol-reducing agents. In Japan a big intervention study using simvastatin (Japan Lipid Intervention Trial, J-LIT) was completed a few years ago [48]. Because all the subjects in J-LIT were administered with simvastatin and the results could not be compared with its own placebo group, another group of investigators selected hyperlipidemic subjects comparable to those of J-LIT [42]. Those recruited were 4,918 hypercholesterolemic (220–299 mg/dl, 5.7–7.7 mmol/l) subjects without the history of AMI but with regular medical checkup at 13 health care centers. Those centers were independent and located all over Japan. The subjects were followed from 1993 to 1999. The proportion of subjects who took lipid-lowering drugs during the first year was 2.6% in the group of the cholesterol levels between 220 and 239 mg/dl and 5.2% in the group between 280 and 299 mg/dl. Those proportions increased to 9.5 and 33.5%, respectively, during the last year of the follow-up. Similarly, the proportion of subjects who received dietary instruction for hypercholesterolemia was 12.7 and 20.6% for those with blood cholesterol levels of 220–239 and 280–299 mg/dl, respectively, and the proportion increased to 27.4 and 40.2%, respectively, at the last year of the study [42]. The subjects were followed under usual care and no intervention was made. During the follow-up period of 6 years, 36 AMI cases were found. Both a Cox hazard model as adjusted for age and sex and a multivariate analysis including blood pressure and diet therapy, that were found significant in the Cox hazard model, showed that the risk of AMI was increased to 2.30- and 2.89-fold, respectively, when dietary instruction was given to subjects at the start of the study (table 3; fig. 4) [42].

The dietary instruction offered to participants of the study above is likely not to have been uniform, because each health care center had their own dietary plans. However, the principal instructions can be summarized as follows: (1) reduce animal meat and increase plant oil; (2) replace butter with soft margarine; (3) reduce foods containing high cholesterol like eggs; (4) increase fiber intake; (5) increase soy and soy products; (6) reduce calories if you are obese; (7) stop smoking. Sometimes fatty fish was recommended because of its EPA and DHA, sometimes not because of its high cholesterol contents. LA was recommended any way.

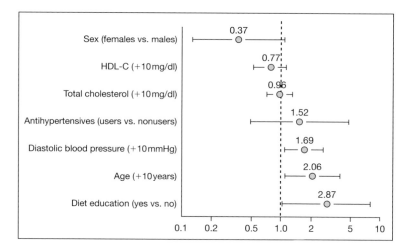

Fig. 4. Multivariate analysis of risk factors for acute myocardial infarction [42]. Adjusted by sex, age, blood pressure and diet. Horizontal bars indicate 95% CI.

All of these three studies (Lyon Heart Study, Helsinki Businessmen Study, control subject study of J-LIT) have one factor in common, namely, they indicate that the recommendation to increase LA consumption is risky for the prevention of CHD.

How Much LA Consumption Is Ideal for the Prevention of CHD?

As we discussed in the section of epidemiological studies, it is likely that 3–4 en% of LA is probably good for the prevention of CHD. Study subjects of 1960s and 1970s did not take much PUFA including ALA. It is, therefore, reasonable to assume that those old reports, which recommended raising P/S ratios, did not always mean increased LA intake. Tables 2 and 3 show the LA intakes of the control or the lowest LA intake groups in terms of en% if available (some are calculated from LA % of the adipose tissue lipids). We propose the LA intake of 3–4 en% as adequate for the prevention of CHD, and as the level which could be achieved safely, because the essential amount is more or less 1 en%.

As shown in figure 1, the trends of CHD incidence and the LA consumption correlate well in Japan. Figure 5 shows a strong association of cardiovascular mortality to the proportion of omega–6 highly unsaturated fatty acids (HUFA) in tissue HUFA (highly unsaturated fatty acids with $\geq$20 carbon chains and $\geq$3 double bonds). These can hardly be reconciled with the idea that increasing LA protects people from CHD.

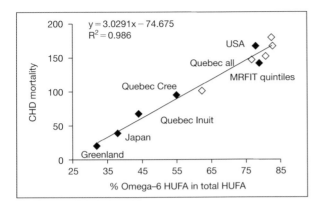

Fig. 5. Coronary heart disease mortality is predicted from tissue omega–6 HUFA. HUFA denotes highly unsaturated fatty acid with carbon chain length of 20 or more and the number of double bonds of 3 or more. Reproduced from reference [12] (by courtesy of Dr. W.E.M. Lands).

The Relationship between LA Intake and Stroke

Iso et al. [49] recently reported on the relationship between the incidence of stroke and the fatty acid composition of stored blood samples. They followed 7,450 Japanese subjects for 6–9 years. The subjects were originally recruited for an epidemiological study to evaluate the incidence of heart disease. During the follow-up period, they found 197 strokes. When calculated with 591 controls, there was a significant inverse correlation between serum LA concentrations and stroke risk (p < 0.05). The total stroke risk was 0.43 (ischemic stroke: 0.33) in the highest quartile compared with that of the lowest quartile [49].

Ischemic stroke was the most prominent subtype of stroke that correlated with LA consumption [49]. However, during the 1960s when the Japanese LA consumption increased rapidly, the incidence of cerebral infarction (nearly equal to ischemic stroke) increased in a parallel manner (fig. 1). Iso et al. [50] have also reported an epidemiological study of stroke incidence in the United States, and found no beneficial effects of LA for stroke prevention. Besides, in the Finnish Mental Hospital Study [36], a sizable increase in LA consumption for 6 years did not decrease the incidence of stroke at all (44 stroke cases in the intervention group and 48 in the control group; table 6). Those facts may suggest that there are important confounding factors in Iso's report, even though statistical adjustments were made for the possible factors [49].

PUFAs are very unstable in the air. Stability decreases with the number of double bonds in the molecule. Consequently, LA is generally assumed to

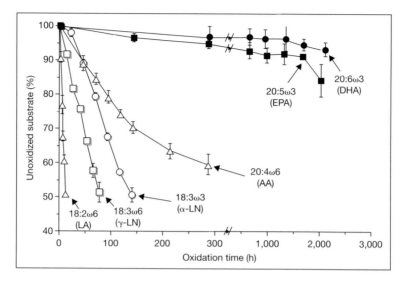

Fig. 6. Changes in the amount of unoxidized PUFAs during oxidation in aqueous emulsion. PUFAs (1 μmol/l) were incubated with Fe^{2+} (1 μmol/l)-ascorbic acid (20 μmol/l) in a phosphate buffer (pH = 7.4) containing 1% Tween 20 at 37°C [51] (by courtesy of Dr. K. Miyashita).

be most stable among the PUFAs because it has only two double bonds. But what would happen in aqueous conditions? Figure 6 beautifully illustrates a completely different story. Miyashita et al. [51] measured the decaying speed of PUFAs in the oxidative aqueous conditions with ascorbic acid and Fe^{2+} as initiators. The more the number of double bonds in PUFA molecules is, the less the vulnerability to oxidative stress is.

Blood samples of the Japanese stroke study [49] were taken from fasting and non-fasting subjects, and were frozen for years before fatty acid analysis. If the decay speed in an aqueous solution is similar to the frozen storage, it might be possible that a certain fraction of subjects, whose blood levels of anti-oxidation vitamins were low, might lose some LA during storage and might be prone to a variety of diseases including stroke. This might have led to an apparent inverse correlation between serum LA and stroke incidence. In fact saturated fatty acid concentrations, which might behave differently from oxidation-vulnerable fatty acids, revealed the opposite correlation to LA [49]. Furthermore, there is always a formidable confounding factor in Japanese (and probably other countries') epidemiological studies with regard to LA; i.e. the attitude of health-consciousness. As written above, Japanese lay people generally believe that LA is good for health. In non-intervention studies, health-conscious people eat, therefore, more LA than others, and the former have better chances to live longer. This confounding factor would often be very difficult to adjust for statistically, unless researchers ask study subjects if they are health-conscious. Despite a negative correlation between the proportion of LA in serum lipids and stroke reported for Japanese subjects [49], one should not start intervention trials along with this observation for the prevention of ischemic stroke before rationale interpretations of the results from other intervention trials [37, 41, 42] were made.

The Relationship between LA Intake and Cancer

Although animal data suggest that LA increases cancer [52], epidemiological data do not support the conclusion drawn from animal experiments in the Western countries [53]. The omega–6/omega–3 ratios of foods are high enough to saturate membrane phospholipids with omega–6 eicosanoid precursors even in the lowest LA intake group in most of the Western countries [12, 52], and a relatively small change in LA intakes does not bring about a significant difference in cancer mortality. Obviously, the increase in the mortality from cancers of the Western type during the past several decades followed the increase in the LA intake in industrialized countries, and some clinical studies support the causal relationship between the LA intake and cancer mortality. Unfortunately, however, there have been no large epidemiological studies reporting the relationship between LA intake and cancer in Japan. The impact of increased LA in the presence of nearly enough omega–3 intakes may be significantly different from the situations in the Western countries.

The Evaluation of LA Changes with Environmental Changes

In the hunter-gatherer ages, LA was an invaluable fatty acid. Famine/starvation, bleeding and infection were the critical points of life and death. Through these points we finally gained the genes to cope with Great Divide. It is unlikely that those genes have changed to any appreciable degree since then. When one got enough LA, he used it as a concentrated source of energy, and part of it would be stored in the adipose tissue for the future starvation (LA is the only PUFA that can be stored in the adipose tissue over 20%; the other PUFAs do not exceed 1% [54]). The rest would be converted to arachidonic acid to be the precursor of eicosanoids. Thromboxane would fight against bleeding; prostaglandins and leukotrienes would fight against parasites through the stimulation of white cells to produce reactive oxygen species. However, bleeding chances and parasites problems have mostly gone long before. In developed countries, there is little use of LA for survival. What we see now is only the negative aspects of excessive LA intake.

Conclusion

During the past several decades, 'increasing the intake of LA while decreasing that of saturated fatty acids' has been the major basis in lipid nutrition for the prevention of CHD. However, the JSLN recommended (2002) that the direction of lipid nutrition should be changed so as to reduce the intake of LA [2]. Here, we attempted to explain from the clinical point of view why LA should be reduced. Furthermore, we proposed that the LA intake of 3–4 en% is adequate for people ingesting omega–3 fatty acids at a level of average Japanese (0.6 en% ALA and 0.5 en% EPA+DHA). However, there is a possibility that reducing the LA intake below 3 en% might accompany ALA (or omega–3 fatty acid) deficiency in those whose fish intake is very low. On the contrary, for those who eat fish regularly, the optimal LA intake might be less than 3 en%.

References

1   Tsuji E, Tsuji K: Fatty acid intake of Japanese people (in Japanese). J Lipid Nutr 1998;7:56–65.
2   http://wwwsoc.nii.ac.jp/jsln/teigenHamazaki02.htm (in Japanese). The home page of the Japan Society for the Lipid Nutrition (April 1, 2003).
3   Health and Welfare Statistics Association: The trend of national hygiene (in Japanese). J Health Welfare Statistics 2002;49(suppl):47–54.
4   Holman RT: Essential Fatty Acid Deficiency. Prog Chem Fat Other Lipids. Pergamon Press, Elmsford, 1968, pp 279–348.
5   Wene JD, Connor WE, DenBesten L: The development of essential fatty acid deficiency in healthy men fed fat-free diets intravenously and orally. J Clin Invest 1975;56:127–134.
6   Naito Y, Iida M, Sato S, et al: Junkanki kensinkoumokukara mita Toshijuuminno shibouni kanrensuru youinno kentou. Nihon Ekigakukai Gakujutsusoukai Kouenshuu 1997, p 98.
7   Uejima H, Okayama A, Sasaki S, et al: Kokuminno daihyosanpuruwo mochiita 14 nenkanno tsuisekikenkyuno gaiyo: 1980 nen junkankishikkan kisochosa tsuisekikenkyu (I). Nihon junkankanrikenkyukyogikai '1980 nen junkanshikkan kisochosa' Tsuisekichosahokokusho 1995, p 752.
8   Shirasaki S: Rokenhokenshinto shiboritsutono kankei – Kokoresuteroruto himanha yokunaika – Nihon Iji Shinpo 1997, No 3831, pp 41–48.
9   Shepherd J, Packard CJ, Patsch JR, et al: Effects of dietary polyunsaturated and saturated fat on the properties of high density lipoproteins and the metabolism of apolipoprotein A-I. J Clin Invest 1978;61:1582–1592.
10   Mattson FH, Grundy SM: Comparison of effects of dietary saturated, monounsaturated, and polyunsaturated fatty acids on plasma lipids and lipoproteins in man. J Lipid Res 1985;26:194–202.
11   Baron JA, Cole BF, Sandler RS, et al: A randomized trial of aspirin to prevent colorectal adenomas. N Engl J Med 2003;348:891–899.
12   Lands WEM: Functional foods in primary prevention or nutraceuticals in secondary prevention? Curr Topics Nutraceut Res 2003;1:113–120.

13 Djoussé L, Pankow JS, Eckfeldt JH, et al: Relation between dietary linolenic acid and coronary artery disease in the National Heart, Lung, and Blood Institute Family Heart Study. Am J Clin Nutr 2001;74:612–619.

14 Franceschi S, Favero A, Decarli A, et al: Intake of macronutrients and risk of breast cancer. Lancet 1996;347:1351–1356.

15 De Stefani E, Deneo-Pellegrini H, Mendilaharsu M, et al: Essential fatty acids and breast cancer: a case-control study in Uruguay. Int J Cancer 1998;76:491–494.

16 Kaaks R, Tuyns AJ, Haelterman M, et al: Nutrient intake patterns and gastric cancer risk: A case-control study in Belgium. Int J Cancer 1998;78:415–420.

17 Bidoli E, La Vecchi C, Montella M, et al: Nutrient intake and ovarian cancer: An Italian case-control study. Cancer Causes Control 2002;13:255–261.

18 de Lorgeril M, Salen P, Martin J-L, et al: Mediterranean dietary pattern in a randomized trial: Prolonged survival and possible reduced cancer rate. Arch Intern Med 1998;158:1181–1187.

19 Bjerve KS: n-3 fatty acid deficiency in man. J Intern Med 1989;225(suppl 1):171–175.

20 Miettinen TA, Naukkarinen V, Huttunen JK, et al: Fatty-acid composition of serum lipids predicts myocardial infarction. Br Med J 1982;285:993–996.

21 Válek J, Hammer J, Kohout M, et al: Serum linoleic acid and cardiovascular death in postinfarction middle-aged men. Atherosclerosis 1985;54:111–118.

22 Wood DA, Riemersma RA, Butler S, et al: Linoleic and eicosapentaenoic acids in adipose tissue and platelets and risk of coronary heart disease. Lancet 1987;i:177–183.

23 Roberts TL, Wood DA, Riemersma RA, et al: Linoleic acid and risk of sudden cardiac death. Br Heart J 1993;70:524–529.

24 Hodgson JM, Wahlqvist ML, Boxall JA, et al: Can linoleic acid contribute to coronary artery disease? Am J Clin Nutr 1993;58:228–234.

25 Pedersen JI, Ringstad J, Almendingen K, et al: Adipose tissue fatty acids and risk of myocardial infarction–a case-control study. Eur J Clin Nutr 2000;54:618–625.

26 Yli-Jama P, Meyer HE, Ringstad J, et al: Serum free fatty acid pattern and risk of myocardial infarction: A case-control study. J Intern Med 2002;251:19–28.

27 Riemersma RA, Wood DA, Butler S, et al: Linoleic acid content in adipose tissue and coronary heart disease. Br Med J 1986;292:1423–1427.

28 Blankenhorn DH, Johnson RL, Mack WJ, et al: The influence of diet on the appearance of new lesions in human coronary arteries. JAMA 1990;263:1646–1652.

29 Tavendale R, Lee AJ, Smith WC, Tunstall-Pedoe H: Adipose tissue fatty acids in Scottish men and women: Results from the Scottish Heart Health Study. Atherosclerosis 1992;94:161–169.

30 Nakamura T, Azuma A, Kuribayashi T, et al: Serum fatty acid levels, dietary style and coronary heart disease in three neighbouring areas in Japan: The Kumihama study. Br J Nutr 2003;89:267–272.

31 Beynen AC, Hermus RJJ, Hautvast JGAJ: A mathematical relationship between the fatty acid composition of the diet and that of the adipose tissue in man. Am J Clin Nutr 1980;33:81–85.

32 Albert CM, Campos H, Stampfer MJ, et al: Blood levels of long-chain n-3 fatty acids and the risk of sudden death. N Engl J Med 2002;346:1113–1118.

33 He K, Rimm EB, Merchant A, et al: Fish consumption and risk of stroke in men. JAMA 2002; 288:3130–3136.

34 Dayton S, Pearce ML, Hashimoto S, et al: A controlled clinical trial of a diet high in unsaturated fat in preventing complications of atherosclerosis. Circulation 1969;40(suppl II):1–63.

35 Leren P: The Oslo diet-heart study: Eleven-year report. Circulation 1970;42:935–942.

36 Miettinen M, Turpeinen O, Karvonen MJ, et al: Effect of cholesterol-lowering diet on mortality from coronary heart-disease and other causes. A twelve-year clinical trial in men and women. Lancet 1972;ii:835–838.

37 Woodhill JM, Palmer AJ, Leelarthaepin B, et al: Low fat, low cholesterol diet in secondary prevention of coronary heart disease. Adv Exp Med Biol 1978;109:317–330.

38 Hjermann I, Velve Byre K, Holme I, et al: Effect of diet and smoking intervention on the incidence of coronary heart disease. Report from the Oslo Study Group of a randomised trial in healthy men. Lancet 1981;ii:1303–1310.

39 Burr ML, Fehily AM, Gilbert JF, et al: Effects of changes in fat, fish, and fibre intakes on death and myocardial reinfarction: Diet and Reinfarction Trial (DART). Lancet 1989;ii:757–761.

40 Frantz ID Jr, Dawson EA, Ashman PL, et al: Test of effect of lipid lowering by diet on cardio-vascular risk. The Minnesota Coronary Survey. Arteriosclerosis 1989;9:129–135.

41 Strandberg TE, Salomaa VV, Naukkarinen VA, et al: Long-term mortality after 5-year multi-factorial primary prevention of cardiovascular diseases in middle-aged men. JAMA 1991;266: 1225–1229.

42 Yoshiike N, Tanaka H, Nihon Shishitsu Kainyusiken Chiikitaisho Tsuisekichosa Group: Nihon Shishitsu Kainyushiken no Chiikitaisho Tsuisekichosa. Lipid 2001;12:281–289.

43 de Lorgeril M, Renaud S, Mamelle N, et al: Mediterranean alpha-linolenic acid-rich diet in secondary prevention of coronary heart disease. Lancet 1994;343:1454–1459.

44 Miettinen TA, Huttunen JK, Naukkarinen V, et al: Multifactorial primary prevention of cardio-vascular diseases in middle-aged men. JAMA 1985;254:2097–2102.

45 Salonen JT, Seppänen K, Nyyssönen K, et al: Intake of mercury from fish, lipid peroxidation, and the risk of myocardial infarction and coronary, cardiovascular, and any death in Eastern Finnish men. Circulation 1995;91:645–655.

46 Guallar E, Sanz-Gallardo MI, van't Veer P, et al: Mercury, fish oils, and the risk of myocardial infarction. N Engl J Med 2002;347:1747–1754.

47 Yoshizawa K, Rimm EB, Morris JS, et al: Mercury and the risk of coronary heart disease in men. N Engl J Med 2002;347:1755–1760.

48 Matsuzaki M, Kita T, Mabuchi H, et al: Large scale cohort study of the relationship between serum cholesterol concentration and coronary events with low-dose simvastatin therapy I Japanese patients with hypercholesterolemia – Primary prevention cohort study of the Japan Lipid Intervention Trial (J-LIT). Circulation J 2002;66:1087–1095.

49 Iso H, Sato S, Umemura U, et al: Linoleic acid, other fatty acids, and the risk of stroke. Stroke 2002;33:2086–2093.

50 Iso H, Rexrode KM, Stampfer MJ, et al: Intake of fish and omega-3 fatty acids and risk of stroke in women. JAMA 2001;285:304–312.

51 Miyashita K, Nara E, Ota T: Oxidative stability of polyunsaturated fatty acids in an aqueous solution. Biosci Biotech Biochem 1993;57:1638–1640.

52 Okuyama H, Kobayashi T, Watanabe S: Dietary fatty acids – the n-6/n-3 balance and chronic elderly diseases. Excess linoleic acid and relative n-3 deficiency syndrome seen in Japan. Prog Lipid Res 1997;35:409–457.

53 Zock PL, Katan MB: Linoleic acid intake and cancer risk: A review and meta-analysis. Am J Clin Nutr 1998;68:142–153.

54 Leaf DA, Connor WE, Barstad L, et al: Incorporation of dietary n-3 fatty acids into the fatty acids of human adipose tissue and plasma lipid classes. Am J Clin Nutr 1995;62:68–73.

Tomohito Hamazaki, Department of Clinical Application
Institute of Natural Medicine, Toyama Medical and Pharmaceutical University
Sugitani, Toyama-shi, Toyama 930–0194 (Japan)
Tel. +81 76 434 7615, Fax +81 76 434 5057, E-Mail hamazaki@ms.toyama-mpu.ac.jp

Simopoulos AP, Cleland LG (eds): Omega–6/Omega–3 Essential Fatty Acid Ratio:
The Scientific Evidence. World Rev Nutr Diet. Basel, Karger, 2003, vol 92, pp 133–151

Omega–6/Omega–3 Polyunsaturated Fatty Acid Ratio and Cancer

Véronique Chajès, Philippe Bougnoux

Nutrition, Croissance, Cancer, INSERM EMI-U 0211,
University François-Rabelais, Tours, France

There is epidemiological support that the long-chain omega–3 polyunsaturated fatty acids (PUFA), including eicosapentaenoic acid (20:5ω3) and docosahexaenoic acid (22:6ω3), which originate from animal marine sources, exert protective effects against common cancers: breast, colon and prostate. Animal studies have generally concluded that omega–6 PUFA, provided by corn and other common seed oils, have tumor-promoting effects at several sites whereas omega–3 PUFA, provided by fish oils, are protective. This oversimplified pattern has been questioned by several experimental data, and several reports support the hypothesis that it may be the balance between omega–6 and omega–3 PUFA, rather than the individual amount of each class of PUFA, which may influence the outcome of cancer.

The evolutionary aspects of diet with emphasis on the ratio of omega–6 to omega–3 fatty acids is reviewed by Simopoulos [1]. In the diet of our ancestors, the ratio of omega–6 to omega–3 essential fatty acids was 1 to 2/1 with higher levels of EPA, DHA and arachidonic acid than today's diet. Today, this ratio is about 4 to 1 in Japan, and varies from 15 to 1 in current United Kingdom and northern Europe to 16.74 to 1 in current United States, indicating that Western diets are depleted in omega–3 fatty acids [2]. The depletion of omega–3 PUFA in Western diets is the consequence of agribusiness, modern agriculture and aquaculture [1]. The high ratio of omega–6 to omega–3 PUFA is the consequence of excessive production of vegetable oils and of the substitution of saturated fat and butter with oils high in omega–6 PUFA to lower serum cholesterol levels, without taking into consideration their adverse effects on overall human metabolism. Only the diet of Crete or the traditional diet of Greece resembles the Paleolithic diets in terms of fiber, antioxidants, saturated fat, monounsaturated fat, and the ratio of omega–6 to omega–3 PUFA is close to

1 to 1 [2]. There is evidence that diet, and specifically a balanced omega–6 to omega–3 PUFA ratio, may have a protective effect on cancer incidence in humans. Since there is competition and opposition of PUFA in the body, research has been conducted to determine the importance of the dietary omega–6/omega–3 fatty acids ratio, rather than the absolute level of individual PUFA, in cancer prevention [3]. A balanced omega–6/ omega–3 ratio in the diet is essential for normal growth and development and should lead to decreases in cardiovascular disease and cancers. This article will focus on the relationship between individual omega–6 PUFA, omega–3 PUFA, and the ratio of omega–6 to omega–3 fatty acids and cancer risk.

Omega–6/Omega–3 Polyunsaturated Fatty Acid Ratio and Breast Cancer

Epidemiology

Breast cancer incidence rates vary greatly across countries. Despite associations of hormonal, reproductive and genetic factors with breast cancer risk, most of the variation in occurrence across populations does not appear to be attributable to established risk factors. Among preventable causes of cancer, dietary factor estimates have been accounting for between 20 and 60% according to the sites [4, 5]. Among dietary factors, fat consumption has received extensive attention. Cohort studies, however, provide little evidence that total fat consumption independent of its energy contribution strongly influences breast cancer risk [6, 7].

Most of the epidemiological studies investigating potential protective effects of omega–3 PUFA on breast cancer risk addressed fish consumption. The preponderance of ecological studies supported an inverse association of fish consumption with breast cancer [8–10]. While case-control studies and cohort studies were less consistent [11–14], several studies reported a significant negative association between estimated consumption of fish or other seafood and postmenopausal disease [15–18]. One study reported no association of overall fish intake with breast cancer risk, but an inverse association of poached fish with breast cancer [19].

In spite of the interest in whether a high intake in omega–3 PUFA and/or a low ratio of omega–6 PUFA to omega–3 PUFA is associated with a decreased risk of breast cancer, most of the studies examined the association between estimated dietary intakes of total saturated, monounsaturated and polyunsaturated fat and breast cancer risk, without data on the type of PUFA [20]. In one case-control study conducted in Finland in a population of 73 breast cancer patients and 55 patients with benign breast disease, the dietary intake of long-chain omega–3 PUFA (eicosapentaenoic acid, docosahexaenoic acid) was significantly lower in breast cancer patients than in controls, particularly in postmenopausal women [21]. In the Netherlands Cohort Study on Diet and Cancer, a significant inverse association was found between dietary alpha-linolenic acid intake and breast cancer risk, whereas no association was found for long-chain omega–3 fatty acids, eicosapentaenoic acid and docosahexaenoic acid [22].

Several population-based studies were undertaken to investigate the relation between omega–3 and omega–6 PUFA composition and breast cancer risk, using biomarkers of past dietary intake of PUFA. In the following studies in which the ratio of PUFA has been taken into account, the ratio of omega–3 to omega–6 PUFA has been considered instead of omega–6 to omega–3 PUFA, and the odds ratio were calculated for the omega–3 to omega–6 PUFA ratio.

A prospective cohort study, aimed at evaluating whether omega–3 PUFA protect against breast cancer, was conducted in Sweden [23]. The omega–3 PUFA levels of phospholipids in prediagnostic sera of 196 women who developed breast cancer were compared to those of 388 referents. No significant association between omega–3 PUFA levels and breast cancer risk was found (table 1). The same lack of association between omega–3 PUFA levels or the ratio of omega–3 to omega–6 PUFA in serum phospholipids and breast cancer risk were already reported in a case-control study conducted in Oslo, Norway, in 87 women who developed breast cancer and 235 women who were free of any diagnosed cancer [24] (table 1). Within a cohort of women in the New York University Women's Health Study, the fatty acid composition of serum phospholipids was determined among 197 breast cancer patients and 197 matched controls [25]. No significant association was found between omega–6 or omega–3 PUFA levels and breast cancer risk, total PUFA (omega–6 and omega–3 PUFA) showed a weak protective effect (table 1). No data on the effect of omega–6 to omega–3 PUFA ratio on breast cancer risk was provided.

The relationship between erythrocyte membrane fatty acids and postmenopausal breast cancer risk was investigated in a prospective study of hormones, diet and breast cancer risk (the ORDET study) conducted in northern Italy. In a cohort of 4,052 postmenopausal women, 71 cases of invasive breast cancer were identified, and two matched control women were randomly selected from among cohort women. A nonsignificant inverse association was found between long-chain omega–3 PUFA levels in erythrocyte membranes and breast cancer risk [26] (table 1). In this study, no data on the relationship between the ratio of omega–6 to omega–3 PUFA and breast cancer risk was provided.

Since adipose tissue has been shown to best reflect dietary exposures for the essential fatty acids (with the linoleic acid, alpha-linolenic acid, and long-chain omega–3 PUFA) [27, 28], several studies used the fatty acid composition

Table 1. Omega–6, omega–3 polyunsaturated fatty acids, omega–6/omega–3 polyunsaturated fatty acids ratio and breast cancer risk

Study type (country)	Population	Biomarker	Exposure	Comparison	Odds ratio (95% CI) p value
Case-control study (Norway) [24]	87 cases/ 235 controls	serum phospholipids	omega–3 PUFA	high vs. low quartile*	0.7 (0.3–1.6)[a] 0.57
			omega–6 PUFA		0.5 (0.2–1.0)[a] 0.05
			omega–3/ omega–6 PUFA		1.0 (0.4–2.1)[a] 0.75
Prospective study (Sweden) [23]	196 cases/ 388 controls	serum phospholipids	omega–3 PUFA	high vs. low quartile*	0.58 (0.27–1.28)[b] 0.281
			omega–6 PUFA		0.91 (0.40–2.06)[b] 0.939
			20:5ω3/20:4ω6		0.88 (0.42–1.86)[b] 0.591
Prospective study (New York, USA) [25]	197 cases/ 197 controls	serum phospholipids	omega–3 PUFA	high vs. low quartile	0.69 (0.35–1.34)[c] 0.30
			omega–6 PUFA		0.70 (0.36–1.36)[c] 0.20
			total PUFA (omega–3 and omega–6)		0.59 (0.31–1.09)[c] 0.09
Prospective study (Italy) [26]	71 cases/ 141 controls	erythrocyte membrane phospholipids	omega–3 PUFA	high vs. low tertile	0.53 (0.26–1.08)[d] 0.07
			omega–6 PUFA		0.49 (0.22–1.06)[d] 0.08
Case-control study (Boston, USA) [29]	postmenopausal women 380 cases/ 176 controls	subcutaneous adipose tissue	20:5ω3	high vs. low quintile	0.7 (0.4–1.1)[e] 0.22
			22:6ω3		1.1 (0.6–1.7)[e] 0.59
			20:4ω6		1.0 (0.6–1.6)[e] 0.60
Case-control study (USA, New York) [30]	154 cases/ 125 controls	subcutaneous and breast adipose tissue	omega–3 PUFA	high vs. low quartile	1.16 (0.58–2.34)[f] 0.40

Study type (country)	Population	Biomarker	Exposure	Comparison	cancer	controls
Case-control study (Finland) [21]	postmenopausal 47 cases/ 20 controls	breast adipose tissue phospholipids	20:5ω3	comparison of percentages	1.48 ± 0.61	1.48 ± 0.58[g]
			22:6ω3		0.56 ± 0.71	1.25 ± 0.93*[g]
			20:4ω6		9.64 ± 2.26	10.95 ± 3.26[g]
	premenopausal 26 cases/ 35 controls		20:5ω3		1.36 ± 0.62	1.14 ± 0.54[g]
			22:6ω3		0.54 ± 0.71	0.97 ± 0.79[g]
			20:4ω6		9.67 ± 2.56	9.58 ± 2.17[g]

Table 1 (continued)

Study type (country)	Population	Biomarker	Exposure	Comparison	Odds ratio (95% CI) p value
Multicentric case-control study (Europe) [31]	all centers pooled; postmenopausal 291 cases/ 351 controls	subcutaneous adipose tissue	long-chain omega–3 PUFA	all centers pooled; high vs. low tertile*	0.93 (0.50–1.70)[h] 0.81
			omega–6 PUFA		1.42 (0.69–2.94)[h] 0.35
			long-chain omega–3/ omega–6 PUFA		0.65 (0.41–1.03)[h] 0.055
Case-control study (France) [32]	241 cases/ 88 controls	breast adipose tissue	omega–3 PUFA	high vs. low tertile*	0.40 (0.17–0.94)[i] 0.001
			omega–6 PUFA		2.29 (0.12–4.69)[i] 0.07
			long-chain omega–3/ omega–6 PUFA		0.33 (0.17–0.66)[i] 0.0002

*Or low versus high tertile of omega–6 to omega–3 PUFA ratio.

[a]The study was based on blood samples provided by the Janus serum bank, initiated in 1973, comprising nearly 500,000 samples from approximately 170,000 donors, who had no diagnosed cancer at the time of blood donation. The case sera have been obtained from women who developed breast cancer up to several years subsequent to blood donation. Three controls, free of any diagnosed cancer, born within 1 year of a case and who had donated blood within 6 months of a case donation, were randomly selected for each case. Analysis was restricted to women who were 55 years and younger (65 cases; 195 controls).

[b]The study has been conducted in three cohort studies in northern Sweden. Two referents were randomly selected for each case from the cohort and matched for age, age of blood sample and sampling center. Results were adjusted for age at menarche, age at full-term pregnancy, number of children, use of hormone-replacement therapy, height and weight.

[c]The study is a part of the prospective New York University Women's Health Study on hormones, diet and cancer. Controls were cohort members free of cancer, randomly selected among those who matched a case by age at recruitment, menopausal status at baseline, date of baseline blood samplings and number of blood sampling before a case's date of diagnosis. Only the baseline blood samples were used for the analysis of fatty acids. Results were adjusted for age at first full-term birth, family history of breast cancer, history of benign breast disease, and total cholesterol.

[d]The study is a part of a prospective study of hormones, diet and breast cancer risk (ORDET) conducted in northern Italy. For each case, two matched control subjects were randomly selected from the cohort. Since body mass index, waist-to-hip ratio, age at menarche, age at first childbirth, age at menopause, months of lactation, parity, and educational level exerted a major confounding effect on the relationship of fatty acids to breast cancer risk, unadjusted odds ratio are presented.

[e]The control group was women with non-proliferative benign breast disease. Results were adjusted for age, alcohol intake, parity, family history of breast cancer, age at first birth, age at menopause, age at menarche, prior history of benign breast disease and weight 5 years before study entry.

[f]The control group was women with benign masses. Results were adjusted for menopausal status and body mass index.

[g]The control group was women with benign breast disease. Values are mean ± SD expressed as percentage of total fatty acids mol%. *$p < 0.01$ (group difference by analysis of covariance with age as covariate).

[h]Controls were randomly selected from populations registries in Germany and Switzerland. Other centers (the Netherlands, Northern Ireland and Spain) drew controls from patient lists of the cases' general practitioners. Results were adjusted for age, body mass index, nulliparity, family history of breast cancer, age exceeding 35 years at first childbirth and study center.

[i]The control group was women with benign breast pathologies. Results were adjusted for age at diagnosis, height, body mass index, menopause, and menopausal status-body mass index interaction.

of adipose tissue samples as a biomarker to investigate the relation between exposure to omega–6 and omega–3 PUFA and breast cancer. The determination of fatty acid profiles in the adipose tissue offers the advantages over question-naire methods of dietary assessment in case-control studies of being free from recall bias and, unlike serum levels of fatty acids, not being potentially altered by recent changes in diet that may occur due to the disease.

In one case-control study conducted in Boston, the association between fatty acid composition of subcutaneous adipose tissue and risk of breast cancer has been investigated in 380 postmenopausal women with newly diagnosed stage I or II breast cancer and 176 postmenopausal women with proliferative breast disease [29]. No consistent associations were found between any of the series of fatty acids or the individual fatty acids (including long-chain omega–3 PUFA) in adipose tissue and breast cancer risk (table 1). The same lack of asso-ciation between omega–3 PUFA in subcutaneous abdomen and breast adipose tissues was observed in another case-control study conducted in New York on 154 women with invasive breast carcinoma and 125 control women with benign breast disease [30] (table 1). In one case-control study conducted in Finland in 73 women with breast cancer and 55 control women with benign breast disease, the level of docosahexaenoic acid (22:6ω3) of phospholipids in breast adipose tissue was significantly lower in cases than in controls among postmenopausal women [21] (table 1). A positive correlation was also found between dietary intake of docosahexaenoic acid and its level in phospholipids of breast adipose tissue. No difference was found in the level of linoleic acid or long-chain omega–6 PUFA in breast adipose tissue between cases and controls (table 1). However, none of these three studies addressed the association of the balance between omega–6 and omega–3 PUFA with breast cancer risk.

In the European Community Multicenter Study on Antioxidants, Myocardial Infarction and Cancer of the breast (EURAMIC), the fatty acid content of adipose tissue from the subcutaneous buttock in postmenopausal breast cancer cases and controls from five European countries (Germany, Switzerland, The Netherlands, Northern Ireland, Spain) was used to explore the hypothesis that omega–3 PUFA levels were inversely associated to breast cancer risk and that the inverse association depended on background levels of omega–6 PUFA [31]. Inverse associations between breast cancer risk and total adipose tissue omega–3 PUFA levels (EPA, DHA and alpha-linolenic acid) appeared in three centers (Zeist, Corelaine, Zurich), with the second and third tertiles having odds ratios below 1.0. However, only one inverse association reached statistical significance (Zurich). In contrast, a positive association was observed in two other centers (Malaga, Berlin), reaching statistical signifi-cance in one center (Malaga). The same patterns of associations were observed when restricting the analyses to long-chain omega–3 PUFA. Alpha-linolenic alone showed a non-significant inverse association with breast cancer risk in two centers (Corelaine, Zurich) and a non-significant positive association in the three other centers. Pooling all centers gave little evidence of an inverse association with breast cancer for total omega–3 PUFA, long-chain omega–3 PUFA and alpha-linolenic acid (table 1). Total omega–6 PUFA (linoleic acid, dihomo-gamma-linolenic acid, arachidonic acid) showed a strong positive association with breast cancer in one center (Malaga). No associations or weak inverse associations were observed in the other centers. Pooling all centers yielded weak evidence of a positive association between omega–6 PUFA and breast cancer risk (table 1). The ratio of total omega–3 PUFA to omega–6 PUFA or the ratio of long-chain omega–3 PUFA to omega–6 PUFA was inversely associated with breast cancer risk in four of five centers. In Spain, the ratio of long-chain omega–3 PUFA to omega–6 PUFA showed a significant inverse association with disease, despite both omega–3 and omega–6 PUFA exhibited significant positive associations with breast cancer. In pooled analyses, the estimated effect for total omega–3 PUFA, long-chain omega–3 PUFA and alpha-linolenic acid were higher when considering them in relation to omega–6 PUFA rather than their absolute levels (table 1). The strongest inverse association with breast cancer was reported for the ratio of long-chain omega–3 PUFA to omega–6 PUFA, with evidence of a dose-response pattern (table 1). In our case-control study conducted in central France, we investigated the association between omega–3 and omega–6 PUFA, the ratio omega–3 PUFA to omega–6 PUFA and the risk of breast cancer [32]. We examined the fatty acid composition in breast adipose tissue from 241 patients with invasive breast carcinoma and from 88 control patients with benign breast disease. We found a positive association between total omega–6 PUFA (but which did not reach statistical significance) and the relative risk of breast cancer and an inverse association between total omega–3 PUFA and the relative risk of breast cancer (table 1). When considering individual levels of omega–6 PUFA, we found a positive association between level of linoleic acid (but which did not reach statistical significance) and the relative risk of breast cancer. Women in the highest tertile of linoleic acid had an odds ratio of 2.31 (95% confidence interval = 1.15−4.67) compared to women in the lowest tertile (p for trend = 0.06). We found no association between arachidonic acid level and the relative risk of breast cancer. Women in the highest tertile of arachidonic acid had an odds ratio of 0.98 (95% confidence interval = 0.42−2.29) compared to women in the lowest tertile (p for trend = 0.32).When considering individual levels of omega–3 PUFA, we found significant inverse associations between levels of alpha-linolenic acid and docosahexaenoic acid and the relative risk of breast cancer. Women in the highest tertile of alpha-linolenic acid had an odds ratio of 0.39

(95% confidence interval = 0.19−0.78) compared to women in the lowest tertile (p for trend = 0.01). Women in the highest tertile of docosahexaenoic acid acid had an odds ratio of 0.31 (95% confidence interval = 0.13−0.75) compared to women in the lowest tertile (p for trend = 0.016). However, the strongest inverse association with breast cancer was found for the ratio of long-chain omega–3 PUFA to omega–6 PUFA (table 1).

This set of data supports the idea that the protective effect of omega–3 PUFA depends on background levels of omega–6 PUFA. Thus, it may be the balance between omega–6 and omega–3 PUFA rather than the individual amount of each class of PUFA which influence the outcome of breast cancer.

Experimental Studies

Studies in animal model of mammary carcinogenesis appeared to support the epidemiological evidence concerning the importance of the ratio of omega–6 to omega–3 PUFA ratio in tumor growth and provided data on the protective role of a ratio of omega–6 to omega–3 PUFA of about 1–2 to 1 against the development of mammary cancer [33]. One of the first studies designed at investigating the effect of omega–6 to omega–3 PUFA ratio on NMU-induced mammary carcinogenesis was reported by Cohen et al. [34]. They varied the proportion of omega–3 PUFA (provided as menhaden oil) to omega–6 PUFA (corn oil) in a high fat diet (23% fat/diet). They found that tumor growth was inhibited only when equal parts of omega–6 and omega–3 PUFA were fed. The same observation has been made in the DMBA-induced mammary tumor model in rats [35]. They reported that the incidence of mammary tumors was suppressed in a group of rats fed fat with a omega–3 to omega–6 PUFA ratio of 0.71 (or omega–6 to omega–3 PUFA ratio = 1.4) when dietary fat comprised 20% of the diet. In another study in which dietary fat comprised 23.5% of the diet, suppression of mammary tumor incidence was observed in a group of rats fed fat with a omega–3 to omega–6 PUFA ratio of 0.91 (or omega–6 to omega–3 PUFA ratio = 1.1) [36]. Sasaki et al. [37] used a 10% fat diet in the DMBA rat model, and varied the proportion of omega–6 and omega–3 PUFA, through mixing coconut oil, safflower oil and fish oil in such a way that the ratio of total PUFA to saturated fatty acids was kept constant. They found that increasing the omega–3 to omega–6 PUFA ratio from 0.01 to 7.8 (0.01; 1.03; 3.96; 7.84) (or decreasing the omega–6 to omega–3 PUFA ratio from 100 to 0.13) did not suppress the incidence nor reduce the latency of mammary tumor development, but even promoted the development of tumors. In this latter study, the total level of dietary fat they used (10%) is lower than those used in the others (about 20%), making difficult direct comparison of the data. Recently, adenoviral stategies were used to introduce the *Caenorhabditis elegans* fat-1 gene encoding an omega–3 fatty acid desaturase into human breast cancer cells in vitro followed by determination of the omega–6/omega–3 fatty acid ratio and growth of the cancer cells [38]. They found that the infection of tumor cells with an adenovirus carrying the fat-1 gene resulted in a high expression of the omega–3 fatty acid desaturase, a change of the omega–6/omega–3 fatty acids ratio in tumor cells from 12.0 to 0.8, along with an induction of cell death and an inhibition of cell proliferation. These data confirm the importance of the ratio of omega–6 PUFA to omega–3 PUFA on the control of tumor growth and indicate a protective role of a ratio of omega–6 to omega–3 PUFA of about 1–2:1 against the development of mammary cancer.

Recent studies have demonstrated that the inhibitory effect of omega–3 PUFA on mammary tumor growth depend upon background levels of omega–6 PUFA and also on antioxidant levels [39]. An experimental study on rats showed that addition of vitamin E to a 15% linseed oil diet rich in alpha-linolenic acid led to an increase in tumor growth compared to controls without vitamin E; whereas addition of pro-oxidant compound (sodium ascorbate/ 2-methyl-1,4-naphthoquinone) led to a decrease in tumor growth [40]. All these data indicate that the inhibitory effects of omega–3 PUFA on tumor growth depends on levels of omega–6 PUFA and antioxidants, and this could account for previously inconsistent results in experimental carcinogenesis.

Omega–6/Omega–3 Polyunsaturated Fatty Acid Ratio and Colorectal Cancer

Epidemiology
Colorectal cancer is one of the most common forms of cancer and related mortality in Western cultures. Besides genetic predisposition, it has been estimated that 90% of the risk of colorectal cancer could be attributed to environmental factors, mostly dietary factors [4]. Although there is a strong positive association between total fat consumption and colorectal cancer risk (reviewed in [41]), there is evidence that omega–3 PUFA, mainly found in fish, exert a protective effect. In an analysis involving 24 European countries, an inverse correlation was found in males between colorectal cancer mortality and current fish intake [42]. Previous epidemiological data were reanalyzed for breast and colorectal cancer, and there was evidence of a protective effect of a high fish intake relative to that of dietary sources of omega–6 fatty acids for both tumor types [43]. These data suggested that fish oil consumption is associated with protection against the promotional effects of animal fat in colorectal carcinogenesis. Several case-control or cohort studies reported inverse associations between fish consumption and risk of colorectal cancer [14, 44–47],

while one prospective study in young men and women reported no association between fish intake and the risk of colon cancer [48]. In the Health Professionals Follow-up Study cohort, the ratio of red meat to the intake of chicken and fish was positively associated with risk of colorectal adenoma [45]. In a prospective study among women, processed meats were associated with increased risk of colon cancer, whereas high intake of fish was related to decreased risk, and the ratio of the intake of red meat to the intake of chicken and fish was particularly strongly associated with increased incidence of colon cancer [44]. These data lend support to existing dietary recommendations to reduce one's intake of meat high in fat (high in omega–3 PUFA) and to substitute fish (high in omega–3 PUFA) and chicken. One cohort study addressed the relationship between specific fatty acids and colorectal cancer risk: no significant association was found for the ω6 PUFA linoleic acid and for omega–3 PUFA, alpha-linolenic acid, EPA and DHA [49]. However, no data on the ratio of omega–6 to omega–3 fatty acids in relation to the risk of colorectal cancer was provided.

Using biomarkers of past dietary intake of PUFA, one ecological study was conducted in 11 centers from 8 European countries and Israel, using adipose tissue PUFA composition as indicator of exposure [50]. No significant association was found between omega–6 PUFA in adipose tissue and colon cancer. A positive correlation was found between omega–3 PUFA levels in adipose tissue and colon cancer ($r = 0.30$), whereas association between estimated fish omega–3 PUFA and colon cancer was weakly negative ($r = -0.19$). No data on the association between omega–6 to omega–3 ratio and colon cancer was provided.

Intervention Studies

There have been several human intervention studies targeted on fish supplementation and colon cancer risk. In a double-blind study, 60 patients with sporadic adenomas received 2.5, 5.1, or 7.7 g of fish oil per day or placebo for 30 days [51]. Significantly reduced rectal proliferation was observed, but only in patients with abnormal baseline rectal proliferation patterns. The effects persisted during long-term supplementation (6 months) in 15 patients with polyps who received 2.5 g fish oil per day [51]. These data indicated that low-dose fish oil supplementation has short-term and long-term normalizing effects on the abnormal rectal proliferation patterns associated with increased risk of colon cancer. Two human studies were carried out in which fish supplementation was given in order to suppress rectal epithelial cell proliferation (intermediate biomarker of cancer risk) and PGE2 biosynthesis [52, 53]. This was achieved when the dietary omega–3/omega–6 PUFA ratio was 0.4 (or omega–6/omega–3 PUFA ratio = 2.5:1) [52], but not with the same absolute level of fish intake (4.4 g omega–3 PUFA/day) and a omega–3/omega–6 PUFA ratio of 0.25 (omega–6/omega–3 PUFA ratio = 4:1) [53]. These results emphasize the importance of dietary omega–6/omega–3 PUFA ratio in determining the effects of fish oil supplementation on parameters of colon cancer.

Experimental Studies
Data from experimental studies on the effect of individual PUFA on human colorectal carcinoma cell lines showed that there is no obvious differential effect between omega–6 and omega–3 PUFA on cell proliferation (reviewed in [54]). In most studies, the essential fatty acids, linoleic acid and alpha-linolenic acid, showed no effect on tumor cell proliferation, while long-chain PUFA, arachidonic acid, EPA and DHA, led to a decrease in cell proliferation or an increase in apoptosis. In addition, DHA supplementation to colon cancer cell line CaCo-2 led to an induction of apoptosis, along with an inactivation of prostaglandin family of genes, lipoxygenases and altered expression of peroxisome proliferators, suggesting that a lipid peroxidation-induced apoptosis by DHA [55]. No data on the effect of the ratio of omega–6 to omega–3 PUFA in relation to cancer cell proliferation was available.

Many experimental studies using in vivo models of colorectal carcinogenesis have been performed to evaluate the effects of diets enriched in omega–3 and omega–6 PUFA. It has been consistently shown that colon tumor enhancing effect of corn oil (omega–6 PUFA) is most prevalent during the postinitiation phase, whereas the tumor inhibiting effect of fish oil (omega–3 PUFA) is observed during both the initiation and postinitiation phases [56]. Comparing fish oil to corn oil, butter or beef tallow, a study reported a lower colon cell proliferation, an intermediate biomarker for colon carcinogenesis, in rats fed fish oils [57]. Among omega–3 PUFA, DHA has been shown to suppress the formation and growth of aberrant crypt foci induced by 2-amino-1-methyl-6-phenylimidazo[4,5-b]pyridine [58] or by azoxymethane [59] in male F344 rats. The effect of various levels of dietary menhaden fish oil plus corn oil fed during the postinitiation phase of colon carcinogenesis was studied in male F344 rats [60]. Experimental diets increased in omega–3 PUFA content from 23.5% corn oil, 17.6% corn oil + 5.9% menhaden oil ratio (omega–6/omega–3 = 2.94), 11.8% corn oil + 11.8% menhaden oil (omega–6/omega–3 = 1) to 5.9% corn oil + 17.6% menhaden oil (omega–6/omega–3 = 0.34). The multiplicity (number of tumors/rat) of colon adenocarcinoma was significantly inhibited only in groups fed the 5.9% corn oil + 17.6% menhaden oil (low omega–6/omega–3 ratio) compared to those fed the 23.5% corn oil [60]. These data indicated that the relative proportions of omega–6 and omega–3 fatty acids in the diet are determinants of the high fat effect.

Omega–6/Omega–3 Polyunsaturated Fatty Acid Ratio and Prostate Cancer

Epidemiology

Interactions between individual genetic susceptibility and the life style background, particularly diet, are responsible for prostate cancer causation. Total fat intake, particularly of animal fats, has been suggested to be associated with a higher incidence and mortality of prostate cancer, although some epidemiological studies have not been consistent in this respect [61].

Recently, much attention has been paid to the roles of omega–6 and omega–3 PUFA as risk and beneficial factors, respectively, for prostate cancer. Although it is suggested that omega–3 PUFA might reduce the risk of prostate cancer, findings from epidemiological studies are still scarce and results are conflicting. In a population-based prospective cohort of 6,272 Swedish men, Terry et al. [49] have recently reported epidemiological data indicating that men who ate no fish had a twofold to threefold higher frequency of prostate cancer than those who ate moderate or high amounts, suggesting a protective effect of fish consumption on prostate cancer risk. However, data from the prospective Health Professionals Follow-up Study conducted in USA showed no association between fish intake and prostate cancer risk [62]. In this study, the authors reported a positive association between dietary intake of alpha-linolenic acid and prostate cancer risk [62]. This is in agreement with results from two case-control studies, one conducted in Uruguay [63], the second conducted in Spain [64], in which they found a positive association between dietary intake of alpha-linolenic acid and risk of prostate cancer. In these studies, no information on long-chain PUFA was available. In a cohort study conducted in the Netherlands, the association between dietary intake of individual fatty acid and prostate cancer risk was investigated [65]. In contrast to results from other studies [62–64], decreased risk of prostate cancer was associated with increasing quintile of alpha-linolenic acid. No associations were found for intake of arachidonic acid, eicosapentaenoic acid, or docosahexaenoic acid. In this study, no data was available on the association concerning the association between the ratio of omega–6 to omega–3 PUFA and prostate cancer risk.

In the prospective Physicians' Health study conducted in USA, a nested case-control study was used to compare fatty acid composition in plasma from 120 men who developed prostate cancer and 120 matched controls who did not: no association was found between one long-chain omega–3 PUFA (20:5 ω3) level in plasma and prostate cancer risk [66]. However, men with elevated levels of plasma alpha-linolenic acid had a twofold to threefold increase in risk of prostate cancer compared with those with low levels (table 2). In a prospective cohort study conducted in Norway (the donor's serum to the Janus serum bank),

Table 2. Omega–3, omega–6 polyunsaturated fatty acids, omega–3/omega–6 polyunsaturated fatty acids ratio and prostate cancer risk

Study type (country)	Population	Biomarker	Exposure	Comparison	Odds ratio (CI 95%) p value		
Nested case-control study (USA) [66]	120 cases/ 120 controls	plasma cholesterol esters	18:3 omega–3	high vs. low quartile	2.14 (0.93–4.93)[a] 0.03		
			20:4 omega–6		1.36 (0.63–2.90)[a] 0.76		
			20:5 omega–3		0.87 (0.41–1.82)[a] 0.81		
Nested case-control study (Norway) [67]	141 cases/ 282 controls	serum phospholipids	omega–3 PUFA	high vs. low quartile	1.1 (0.6–2.1)[b] 0.9		
			18:2ω6/18:3ω3		0.3 (0.2–0.8)[b] 0.01		
			20:4ω6/20:5ω3		0.8 (0.4–1.5)[b] 0.05		
Case-control study (USA) [68]	89 cases/ 38 controls	erythrocyte membranes	18:3 omega–3	high vs. low quartile	1.69 (0.54–5.26)[c] 0.23		
			20:5 omega–3		0.74 (0.23–2.33)[c] 0.12		
			22:6 omega–3		0.36 (0.10–1.27)[c] 0.11		
			18:2 omega–6		3.54 (1.0–12.53)[c] 0.04		
Case-control study (USA) [68]	89 cases/ 38 controls	adipose tissue	18:3 omega–3	high vs. low quartile	2.73 (0.70–10.61)[c] 0.18		
			20:5 omega–3		0.54 (0.18–1.62)[c] 0.12		
			22:6 omega–3		1.11 (0.30–4.14)[c] 0.46		
			18:2 omega–6		2.47 (0.66–9.26)[c] 0.08		
Case-control study (USA) [69]	67 cases/ 156 controls	erythrocyte membranes	18:3 omega–3	high vs. low quartile	2.6 (1.1–5.8)[d] 0.01		
			total omega–3 PUFA		1.1 (0.5–2.5)[d] 0.78		
			total omega–6 PUFA		2.3 (1.0–5.4)[d] 0.10		
Case-control study (Korea) [70]	19 cases/ 24 controls with benign breast disease/21 controls without cancer	serum phospholipids		1[e]	2[e]	3[e]	
			omega–3 PUFA	15.22 ± 4.56	11.98 ± 3.29	10.44 ± 2.45[f]	
			omega–6 PUFA	17.20 ± 2.91	16.79 ± 3.08	3.46 ± 3.46[f]	
			omega–3/ omega–6 PUFA	0.89 ± 0.21	0.71 ± 0.12	0.50 ± 0.14[f]	

Table 2 (continued)

Study type (country)	Population	Biomarker	Exposure	Comparison		Odds ratio (CI 95%) p value
				1[g]	2[g]	
Case-control study (Greece) [71]	36 cases/ 35 controls	prostatic tissue	omega–3 PUFA	2.76 ± 0.87	1.84 ± 0.79[h]	
			omega–6 PUFA	18.93 ± 3.53	15.72 ± 3.17[h]	
			omega–3/ omega–6 PUFA	0.14 ± 0.03	0.11 ± 0.03[h]	

[a]Part of the Physician's Health Study, on a population of 14,916 US male physicians who provided plasma samples. 120 men who later developed prostate cancer and 120 controls who did not. Unadjusted estimated relative risks of prostate cancer by level of baseline plasma cholesterol fatty acids.

[b]The study was carried out as a nested case-control study among men with no known prostate cancer at the time of blood sampling. The population contributed serum to the Janus serum bank in Norway. Controls were matched to cases by country, age, and date of blood sample.

[c]Cases were recruited from a university-based urology outpatient clinic and had confirmation of a prostate cancer diagnosis within one year of entry into the study. Controls were free of prostate cancer, recruited from the same clinic over the same period and had a prostate biopsy or a prostatectomy specimen that was free of prostate cancer. The base model included race and age as covariates.

[d]Cases were newly diagnosed with primary adenocarcinoma of the prostate. Controls were selected in the population such as they have a similar age distribution as the cases. Results were adjusted for age.

[e]1 = 21 patients without evidence of benign or malignant prostatic disease; 2 = 24 subjects with benign prostatic hyperplasia; 3 = 19 patients with prostate cancer.

[f]Mean values ± SD; comparison among the three groups was made by one-way analysis of variation (ANOVA); $p < 0.05$.

[g]1 = 35 patients with benign hyperplasia; 2 = 23 patients with prostate cancer.

[h]Mean values ± SD; $p < 0.01$.

fatty acid levels determined in serum before diagnosis were compared between subjects who later developed prostate cancer and donors without prostate cancer [67]. They found no significant association between the risk effect and total omega–3 PUFA (table 2) and total omega–6 PUFA (odds ratio for highest versus lowest quartile 0.7, 95% CI 0.3–1.3, p for trend 0.1). In agreement to the findings of Gann et al., increased risk of prostate cancer was found with increasing quartile of alpha-linolenic acid (odds ratio for highest versus lowest quartile 2.0, 95% CI 1.1–3.6, p for trend 0.03). In this study, a negative association between the ratio of linoleic to alpha-linolenic acid or arachidonic acid/ eicosapentaenoic acid and the risk of prostate cancer was found (table 2).

In a case-control study conducted in USA in a population of 89 patients with prostate cancer and 38 control subjects, levels of omega–3 PUFA in erythrocytes membranes and adipose tissue were not associated to prostate cancer risk [68] (table 2). A high level of linoleic acid, both in erythrocyte membranes and adipose tissue, was associated to an increased risk of prostate cancer (table 2). In agreement with this finding, in a case-control study conducted in USA in a population of 67 incident prostate cancer cases and 156 population-based controls, positive associations were observed between cancer risk and levels of linoleic acid (odds ratio for highest versus lowest quartile 2.1, 95% CI 0.9–4.8, p for trend 0.05) and total omega–6 PUFA (table 2), suggesting that omega–6 PUFA increased risk of prostate cancer [69]. Increased risk of prostate cancer was associated with increased level of alpha-linolenic acid (table 2). No significant association was found between total omega–3 PUFA and prostate cancer risk (table 2). In all these studies, no data was available on the association between omega–6 to omega–3 ratio and prostate cancer risk.

Two studies investigated the association between the ratio of omega–3 to omega–6 PUFA and prostate cancer risk. In a case-control study conducted in Korea, serum omega–6 and omega–3 PUFA levels were determined in 21 subjects without benign or malignant prostatic disease, 24 patients with benign prostatic hyperplasia and 19 patients with prostate cancer [70]. They found that omega–3 to omega–6 PUFA ratio of patients with cancer was lower than that of control subjects and patients with benign prostatic disease was ranked between them (table 2). In a case-control study conducted in Greece in a population of 35 patients with benign hyperplasia of the prostate and 36 patients with prostatic malignancy, there was a significantly reduced omega–3 to omega–6 PUFA ratio in prostatic tissue in prostate cancer than in benign hyperplasia group [71] (table 2). These data may indicate that the ratio of omega–6 to omega–3 PUFA, rather than the individual amount of fatty acids, may be of importance to influence the outcome of prostate cancer. However, conflicting findings on the effect of specific fatty acids (specifically alpha-linolenic acid) are provided and more studies with extensive information on the ratio of omega–6 to omega–3 PUFA are needed to clarify the role in prostate carcinoma etiology.

Experimental Studies

Few experimental studies on PUFA and prostate cancer are available due, in part, to the difficulty of chemically inducing prostate cancer in rodents. Growth of transplanted DU-145 human prostatic cancer cells in nude mice was reduced when dietary corn oil (23.52%) was replaced by fish oil (20.52% + 3% corn oil) [36]. In vitro studies on diverse prostate cancer cell lines have provided conflicting results. On human metastatic PC-3, LNCaP and TSU prostate cell lines, supplementation with linoleic acid (1–100 ng/ml) led to a stimulation of proliferation, and supplementation with alpha-linolenic acid, or eicosapentaenoic acid, at low concentrations led to a promotion [72]. In contrast, another study reported an inhibitory effect of docosahexaenoic acid and eicosapentaenoic acid on androgen-mediated cell growth in LNCaP prostate cancer cells [73]. In PC-3 human prostate cancer cells, a study showed that linoleic acid and arachidonic acid stimulate tumor growth while the omega–3 fatty acid, eicosapentaenoic acid, inhibited growth [74]. To date, no work has been done in experimental systems of prostate carcinogenesis to study the effects of varying the amount of omega–3 PUFA relative to omega–6 PUFA intake on tumor growth.

Conclusion

Epidemiological and experimental studies suggest that the most important aspect of PUFA in the prevention of cancer is the ratio of omega–6 to omega–3 PUFA rather than the absolute concentration of either. In the Western diets, the omega–6/omega–3 PUFA ratio is 15/1 to 16.7/1. The scientific evidence is strong for decreasing the omega–6 PUFA intake and increasing the omega–3 PUFA intake in order to provide a ratio of omega–6 to omega–3 PUFA of about 1–2:1, as found in the Cretan diet. Epidemiological and experimental research indicates that a ratio of about 1:1–2:1 has the most protective effect against the development and growth of mammary and colon cancers. Less information is available on the role of omega–3 PUFA on prostate cancer, and findings are conflicting. Specifically, the positive association between dietary intake of alpha-linolenic acid and prostate cancer risk remains to be clarified. There is now a need for the initiation of intervention trials that will test the efficacy of this specific pattern in the prevention of cancer. Experimental studies targeted on the omega–6 to omega–3 PUFA ratio in relation to antioxidant levels should be also addressed. Finally, data provided in such future studies could provide information concerning the use of omega–3 PUFA as chemopreventive agents.

References

1   Simopoulos AP: The importance of the ratio of omega–6/omega–3 essential fatty acids. Biomed Pharmacother 2002;21:495–505.
2   Simopoulos AP: The Mediterranean diets: What is so special about the diet of Greece? The scientific evidence. J Nutr 2001;131:3065S–3073S.
3   Rose DP, Connolly JM: Omega–3 fatty acids as cancer chemopreventive agents. Pharmacol Ther 1999;83:217–244.
4   Doll R, Peto R: The causes of cancer: Quantitatives estimates of avoidable risks of cancer in the United States today. J Natl Cancer Inst 1981;66:1191–1308.
5   Doll R: The lessons of life: Keynote address to the nutrition and cancer conference. Cancer Res 1992;52:2024s–2029s.
6   Willett WC, Hunter DJ, Stampfer MJ, et al: Dietary fat and fiber in relation to risk of breast cancer. JAMA 1992;268:2037–2044.
7   Hunter DJ, Spiegelman D, Adami H, et al: Cohort studies of fat intake and the risk of breast cancer – A pooled analysis. N Engl J Med 1996;334:356–361.

8   Kaizer L, Boyd NF, Kriukov V, Tritchler D: Fish consumption and breast cancer risk: An ecological study. Nutr Cancer 1989;12:61–68.

9   Sasaki S, Horacsek M, Kestleloot H: An ecological study of the relationship between dietary intake and breast cancer mortality. Prev Med 1993;22:187–202.

10   Guo W, Chow W, Zheng W, et al: Diet, serum markers and breast cancer mortality in China. Jpn J Cancer Res 1994;85:572–577.

11   Ingram DM, Nottage E, Roberts T: The role of diet in the development of breast cancer: A case-control study of patients with breast cancer, benign epithelial hyperplasia and fibrocystic disease of the breast. Br J Cancer 1991;64:187–191.

12   Toniolo P, Riboli E, Shore R, Pasternack BS: Consumption of meat, animal products, protein, and fat and risk of breast cancer: A prospective cohort study in New York. Epidemiology 1994;5:391–397.

13   Yuan JM, Wang QS, Ross RK, et al: Diet and breast cancer in Shangai and Tianjin, China. Br J Cancer 1995;71:1353–1358.

14   Fernandez E, Chatenoud L, La Vecchia C, Negri E, Franceschi S: Fish consumption and cancer risk. Am J Clin Nutr 1999;70:85–90.

15   Malik IA, Sharif S, Malik F, et al: Nutritional aspects of mammary carcinogenesis: A case-control study. J Park Med Assoc 1993;43:118–120.

16   Landa MC, Frago N, Tres A: Diet and the risk of breast cancer in Spain. Eur J Cancer Prev 1994; 3:313–320.

17   Hirose K, Kazuo T, Hamajima N, et al: A large-scale, hospital-based case-control study of risk factors of breast cancer according to menopausal status. Jpn J Cancer Res, 1995;86:146–154.

18   Braga C, La Vecchia C, Negri E, Franceschi S, Parpinel M: Intake of selected foods and nutrients and breast cancer risk: An age- and menopause-specific analysis. Nutr Cancer 1997;28:258–263.

19   Vatten LJ, Solvoll K, Løken EB: Frequency of meat and fish intake and risk of breast cancer in a prospective study of 14,500 Norwegian women. Int J Cancer 1990;46:12–15.

20   Smith-Warner SA, Spiegelman D, Adami HO, et al: Types of dietary fat and breast cancer: A pooled analysis of cohort studies. Int J Cancer 2001;92:767–774.

21   Zhu ZR, Ågren S, Männistö S, et al: Fatty acid composition of breast adipose tissue in breast cancer patients and in patients with benign breast disease. Nutr Cancer 1995;24:151–160.

22   Voorrips L, Brants H, Kardinaal A, Hiddink G, van den Brandt P: Intake of conjugated linoleic acid, fat, and other fatty acids in relation to postmenopausal breast cancer: The Netherlands Cohort Study on Diet and Cancer. Am J Clin Nutr 2002;76:873–882.

23   Chajès V, Hultén K, Van Kappel AL, Winkvist A, Kaaks R, Hallmans G, Lenner P, Riboli E: Fatty acid composition in serum phospholipids and risk of breast cancer: An incident case-control study in Sweden. Int J Cancer 1999;83:585–590.

24   Vatten LJ, Bjerve KS, Andersen A, Jellum E: Polyunsaturated fatty acids in serum phospholipids and risk of breast cancer: A case-control study from the Janus Bank in Norway. Eur J Cancer 1993; 29A:532–538.

25   Saadatian-Elahi M, Toniolo P, Ferrari P, Goudable J, Akhmedkhanov A, Zeleniuch-Jacquotte A, Riboli E: Serum fatty acids and risk of breast cancer in a nested case-control study of the New York University Women's Health Study. Cancer Epidemiol Bio Prev 2002;11:1353–1360.

26   Pala V, Krogh V, Muti P, Chajès V, Riboli E, Micheli A, Saadatian M, Sieri S, Berrino F: Erythrocyte membrane fatty acids and subsequent breast cancer: A prospective Italian study. J Natl Cancer Inst 2001;93:1088–1095.

27   London SJ, Sacks FM, Caesar J, et al: Fatty acid composition of subcutaneous adipose tissue and diet in postmenopausal US women. Am J Clin Nutr 1991;54:340–345.

28   Kohlmeier L, Kohlmeier M: Adipose tissue as a medium for epidemiologic exposure assessment. Environ Hlth Perspect 1995;103:99–106.

29   London SJ, Sacks FM, Stampfer MJ, Henderson IC, et al: Fatty acid composition of the subcutaneous adipose tissue and risk of proliferative benign breast disease and breast cancer. J Natl Cancer Inst 1993;85:785–793.

30   Petrek JA, Hudgins LC, Levine B, Ho M, Hirsch J: Breast cancer risk and fatty acids in the breast and abdominal adipose tissues. J Natl Cancer Inst 1994;86:53–56.

31   Simonsen N, Van't Veer P, Strain JJ, Martin-Moreno JM, et al: Adipose tissue omega–3 and omega–6 fatty acid content and breast cancer in the EURAMIC study. Am J Epidemiol 1998;147:342–352.

32   Maillard V, Bougnoux P, Ferrari P, Jourdan ML, Pinault M, Lavillonnière F, Body G, Le Floch O, Chajès V: N-3 and n-6 fatty acids in breast adipose tissue and relative risk of breast cancer in a case-control study in Tours, France. Int J Cancer 2002;98:78–83.

33   Cowing BE, Saker KE: Polyunsaturated fatty acids and epidermal growth factor receptor/mitogen-activated protein kinase signaling in mammary cancer. J Nutr 2001;131:1125–1128.

34   Cohen LA, Chen-Backlund JY, Sepkovic DW, Sugie S: Effect of varying proportions of dietary menhaden and corn oil on experimental rat mammary tumor promotion. Lipids 1993;28:449–456.

35   Ip C, Ip MM, Sylvester P: Relevance of trans fatty acids and fish oils in animal tumorigenesis studies. Prog Clin Biol Res 1986;222:283–294.

36   Karmali RA, Doshi RU, Adams L, Choi K: Effect of n-3 fatty acids on mammary tumorigenesis; in Samuelsson B, Paoletti R, Ramwell PW (eds): Advances in Prostaglandin, Thromboxane, and Leukotriene Research. New York, Raven Press, 1987, vol 17, pp 886–889.

37   Sasaki T, Kobayashi Y, Shimizu J, Wada M, In'nami S, Kanke Y, Takita T: Effects of dietary n-3 to n-6 polyunsaturated fatty acid ratio on mammary carcinogenesis in rats. Nutr Cancer 1998;30: 137–143.

38   Ge Y, Chen Z, Kang ZB, Cluette-Brown J, Laposata M, Kang JX: Effects of adenoviral gene transfer of C. elegans n-3 fatty acid desaturase on the lipid profile and growth of human breast cancer cells. Anticancer Res 2002;22:537–543.

39   Bougnoux P: n-3 polyunsaturated fatty acids and cancer. Curr Opin Clin Nutr Metab Care 1999; 2:121–126.

40   Cognault S, Jourdan ML, Germain E, Pitavy R, Morel E, Durand G, Bougnoux P, Lhuillery C: Effect of an alpha-linolenic acid-rich diet on rat mammary tumor growth depends on the dietary oxidative status. Nutr Cancer 2000;36:33–41.

41   Boutron MC, Wilpart M, Faivre J: Diet and colorectal cancer. Eur J Cancer Prev 1991;1:13–20.

42   Caygill CPJ, Hill MJ: Fish, n-3 fatty acids and human colorectal and breast cancer mortality. Eur J Cancer Prev 1995;4:329–332.

43   Caygill CP, Charlett A, Hill MJ: Fat, fish, fish oil and cancer. Br J Cancer 1996;74:159–164.

44   Willett WC, Stampfer MJ, Colditz GA, Rosner BA, Speize FE: Relation of meat, fat, and fiber intake to the risk of colon cancer in a prospective study among women. N Engl J Med 1990;323: 1664–1672.

45   Giovannucci E, Rimm EB, Stampfer MJ, Colditz GA, Ascherio A, Willett WC: Intake of fat, meat, and fiber in relation to risk of colon cancer in men. Cancer Res 1994;54:2390–2397.

46   Franceschi S, Favero A, La Vecchia C, et al: Food groups and risk of colorectal cancer in Italy. Int J Cancer 1997;72:56–61.

47   Kato I, Akhmedkhanov A, Koenig K, Toniolo P, Shore RE, Riboli E: Prospective study of diet and female colorectal cancer: The New York University Women's Health Study. Nutr Cancer 1997;28: 276–281.

48   Gaard M, Tretli S, Løken EB: Dietary factors and risk of colon cancer: A prospective study of 50,535 young Norwegian men and women. Eur J Cancer Prev 1996;5:445–454.

49   Terry P, Lichenstein P, Feychting M, Ahlbom A, Wolk A: Fatty fish consumption and risk of prostate cancer. Lancet 2001;357:1764–1766.

50   Bakker N, van't Veer P, Zock PL: The EURAMIC study Group. Adipose fatty acids and cancers of the breast, prostate and colon: An ecological study. Int J Cancer 1997;72:587–591.

51   Anti M, Armeleo F, Marra G, Percesepe A, Bartoli GM, Palozza P, Parrella P, Canetta C, Gentiloni N, De Vitis I, et al: Effects of different doses of fish oil on rectal cell proliferation in patients with sporadic colonic adenomas. Gastroenterology 1994;107:1709–1718.

52   Bartram HP, Gostner A, Scheppach W, Reddy BS, Rao CV, Dusel G, Richter F, Richter A, Kasper H: Effects of fish oil on rectal cell proliferation mucosal fatty acids, and prostaglandin E2 release in healthy subjects. Gastroenterology 1993;105:1317–1322.

53   Bartram HP, Gostner A, Reddy BS, Rao CV, Scheppach W, Dusel G, Richter A, Richter F, Kasper H: Missing antiproliferative effect of fish oil on rectal epithelium in healthy volunteers consuming a high-fat diet: Potential role of the n-3:n-6 fatty acid ratio. Eur J Cancer Prev 1995;4:231–237.

54   Dommels YEM, Alink GM, van Bladeren PJ, van Ommen B: Dietary n-6 and n-3 polyunsaturated fatty acids and colorectal carcinogenesis: Results from cultured colon cells, animal models and human studies. Envir Toxicol Pharmacol 2003; in press.

55   Narayanan BA, Narayanan NK, Reddy BS: Docosahaenoic acid regulated genes and transcription factors inducing apoptosis in human colon cancer cells. Int J Oncol 2001;19:1255–1262.

56   Reddy BS, Burill C, Rigotty J: Effects of diets high in omega–3 and omega–6 fatty acids on initiation and post initiation stages of colon carcinogenesis. Cancer Res 1991;51:487–491.

57   Kim DY, Chung KH, Lee JH: Stimulatory effects of high-fat diets on colon cell proliferation depend on the type of dietary fat and site of colon. Nutr Cancer 1998;30:118–123.

58   Takahashi M, Totsuka Y, Masuda M, Fukuda K, Oguri A, Yazawa K, Sugimura T, Wakabayashi K: Reduction in formation of 2-amino-1-methyl-6-phenylimidazo[4,5-b]pyridine (PhIP)-induced aberrant crypt foci in the rat colon by docosahexaenoic acid (DHA). Carcinogenesis 1997;18: 1937–1941.

59   Takahashi M, Fukutake M, Isoi T, Fukuda K, Sato H, Yazawa K, Sugimura T, Wakabayashi K: Suppression of azoxymethane-induced rat colon carcinoma development by a fish oil component, docosahexaenoic acid (DHA). Carcinogenesis 1997;18:1337–1342.

60   Reddy BS, Sugie S: Effect of different levels of omega–3 and omega–6 fatty acids on azoxymethane-induced colon carcinogenesis in F344 rats. Cancer Res 1988;48:6642–6647.

61   Shirai T, Asamoto M, Takahashi S, Imaida K: Diet and prostate cancer. Toxicology 2002;181–182: 89–94.

62   Giovannucci E, Rimm EB, Colditz GA, Stampfer MJ, Ascherio A, Chute CC, Willett WC: A prospective study of dietary fat and risk of prostate cancer. J Natl Cancer Inst 1993;85:1571–1579.

63   De Stéfani E, Deneo-Pellegrini H, Boffetta P, Ronco A, Mendilaharsu M: α-linolenic acid and risk of prostate cancer: A case-control study in Uruguat. Cancer Epidemiol Bio Prev 2000;9:335–338.

64   Ramon JM, Bou R, Romea S, Alkiza ME, Jacas M, Ribes J, Oromi J: Dietary fat intake and prostate cancer risk: A case-control study in Spain. Cancer Causes Control 2000;11:679–685.

65   Schuurman AG, Van den Brandt PA, Dorant E, Brants HAM, Goldbohm RA: Association of energy and fat intake with prostate carcinoma risk. Results from the Netherlands Cohort Study. Cancer 1999;86:1019–1027.

66   Gann PH, Hennekens CH, Sacks FM, Grodstein F, Giovannucci EL, Stampfer MJ: Prospective study of plasma fatty acids and risk of prostate cancer. J Natl Cancer Inst 1994;86:281–286.

67   Harvei S, Bjerve KS, Tretli S, Jellum E, Robsahm TE, Vatten L: Prediagnostic level of fatty acids in serum phospholipids: omega–3 and omega–6 fatty acids and the risk of prostate cancer. Int J Cancer 1997;71:545–551.

68   Godley PA, Campbell MK, Gallagher P, Martinson FE, Mohler JL, Sandler RS: Biomarkers of essential fatty acid consumption and risk of prostatic carcinoma. Cancer Epidemiol Bio Prev 1996;5:889–895.

69   Newcomer LM, King IB, Wicklund KG, Standford JL: The association of fatty acids with prostate cancer risk. Prostate 2001;47:262–268.

70   Yang YJ, Lee SH, Hong SJ, Chung BC: Comparison of fatty acid profiles in the serum of patients with prostate cancer and benign prostatic hyperplasia. Clin Biochem 1999;32:405–409.

71   Mamalakis G, Kafatos A, Kalogeropoulos N, Andrikopoulos N, Daskalopulos G, Kranidis A: Prostate cancer vs hyperplasia: Relationships with prostatic and adipose tissue fatty acid composition. Prostaglandins Leukotrienes Essential Fatty Acids 2002;66:467–477.

72   Pandalai PK, Pilat MJ, Yamazaki K, Naik H, Pienta KJ: The effects of omega–3 and omega–6 fatty acids on in vitro prostate cancer growth. Anticancer Res 1996;16:815–820.

73   Chung BH, Mitchell SH, Zhang JS, Young CY: Effects of docosahexaenoic acid and eicosapentaenoic acid on androgen-mediated cell growth and gene expression in LNCaP prostate cancer cells. Carcinogenesis 2001;22:1201–1206.

74   Hughes-Fulford M, Chen Y, Tjandrawinata RR: Fatty acid regulates gene expression and growth of human prostate cancer PC-3 cells. Carcinogenesis 2001;22:701–707.

Véronique Chajès, MD
Nutrition, Crossance, Cancer, INSERM EMI-U 0211
University François-Rabelais, 2, bis Bd Tonnellé, F–37032 Tours (France)
Tel. +33 2 4736 6179, Fax +33 2 4736 6226, E-Mail chajes@igr.fr

Simopoulos AP, Cleland LG (eds): Omega–6/Omega–3 Essential Fatty Acid Ratio:
The Scientific Evidence. World Rev Nutr Diet. Basel, Karger, 2003, vol 92, pp 152–168

....

Omega–6/Omega–3 Fatty Acids and Arthritis

Leslie G. Cleland, Michael J. James, Susanna M. Proudman

Rheumatology Unit, Royal Adelaide Hospital, Adelaide, S.A., Australia

Arthritis is a generic term that refers to afflictions of joints. Inflammation is involved in almost all forms of arthritis, including those in which the primary problem is usually described as 'degenerative' (osteoarthritis). The presence of inflammation implies mediation of symptoms by inflammatory lipids and proteins as well as structural damage by proteolytic enzymes. The latter degrade structural proteins within cartilage and supportive structures around joints.

Polyunsaturated fatty acids of both omega–6 and omega–3 classes are essential requirements in the diet of vertebrates, which lack the desaturase enzymes necessary to generate these fatty acids de novo. Lands et al. [1] have described the quantitative relationships between omega–6 and omega–3 polyunsaturated fatty acids (PUFA) and highly unsaturated fatty acids (HUFA) in the diet and in the tissues. Differences in culturally determined dietary patterns and individual food choices can generate levels of omega–6 HUFA as a proportion of total plasma phospholipid HUFA in free living subjects that range from 15 to 90%. Most of this omega–6 HUFA is arachidonic acid (AA) (~80%) and proportions of tissue phospholipids HUFA correlate closely with plasma phospholipid HUFA. Furthermore, omega–6 and omega–3 HUFA are located in the *sn*2 position of phospholipids, where they compete for incorporation and release and where their levels are related reciprocally. HUFA are released by phospholipase A_2 for metabolism by the eicosanoid forming enzymes, such as cyclooxygenases-1 and -2 (COX-1 and COX-2) and 5-lipoxygenase. Since the omega–3 HUFA, eicosapentaenoic acid (EPA) and docosahexaenoic acid (DHA), act as competitive inhibitors of conversion of AA to pro-inflammatory eicosanoids, dietary habits may have a considerable influence on an individual's propensity to become and remain inflamed. This may find expression in low grade persistent vessel wall inflammation (atherosclerosis), which remains essentially occult until revealed by

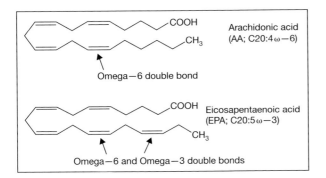

Fig. 1. Structures of the 20-carbon omega–6 and omega–3 fatty acids.

a 'vascular accident', such as a heart attack or stroke, to which it predisposes. In the case of joints, inflammation tends to be symptomatic intrinsically, due to the special property of joints to act as the pivot for movements that are integral to everyday activities. Since movement inevitably involves compressive and traction stresses and the synovium is richly innervated, the nociceptive effects of inflammation will readily translate into pain experience in joints. This tendency is compounded by the tamponade effect that occurs within joints that are swollen by an inflammatory exudate [2]. Thus, in contrast to vascular disease, inflammation in joints causes overt discomfort and interferes with everyday activities at an early stage. However, like vascular inflammation, the long-term effects of inflammatory tissue damage are irreversible tissue damage and functional failure.

PGE$_2$: Its Nociceptive Effect and Synthesis

A dominant symptom of arthritis is pain and associated sensory experiences such as stiffness and loss of function. In the presence of joint pain some degree of avoidance of use is usual. PGE$_2$ is nociceptive and an important mediator of the pain associated with inflammation [3]. This mediator is formed as a result of a multistep metabolic process that involves release of AA (20:4omega–6) from cell membrane phospholipids (fig. 1, 2). COX acts on AA to form the unstable intermediate, PGH$_2$, which in turn is a substrate for terminal synthases, such as PGE synthase which produces PGE$_2$. However, PGH$_2$ is also a substrate for synthases that produce other eicosanoids such as thromboxane (TX) A$_2$. While TXA$_2$ does not appear to be nociceptive, it is an important upregulator of synthesis of the inflammatory cytokines, tumor necrosis factor-α (TNFα) and interleukin-1β (IL-1β) [4], which have been implicated in the long-term tissue damage seen in inflammatory diseases such

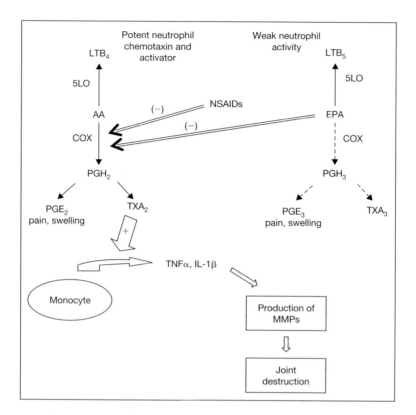

Fig. 2. Metabolism of omega–6 and omega–3 20-carbon fatty acids. 5LO = 5-Lipoxygenase; COX = cyclooxygenase-1 or -2; LTB = leukotriene B; TXA = thromboxane A; PGE = prostaglandin E; NSAIDs = non-steroidal anti-inflammatory drugs. ⟶ Metabolism; ⇢ poor metabolism; (–) inhibition.

as rheumatoid arthritis (RA) [5]. With regard to inflammatory cytokine synthesis, PGE_2 has the opposite effect to that of TXA_2 in that it inhibits TNFα and IL-1β synthesis [4]. Inhibition of COX has long been a target for pharmacotherapy designed to reduce that component of pain from inflammation that is mediated or amplified by PGE_2. The kinetic properties of the respective terminal synthases are such that an increased ratio of TXA_2/PGE_2 synthesis is an unintended consequence of the incomplete pharmacological inhibition of COX activity [6].

Dietary Omega–3 Fats and Eicosanoid Synthesis

Dietary omega–3 fats are competitors with homologous omega–6 fats for remodelling to HUFA and for incorporation into cell membranes.

Table 1. Relative potencies of omega–6 and omega–3 eicosanoids

Fatty acid	Eicosanoid	Action	Omega–6/omega–3[1]
AA/EPA omega–6/omega–3	LTB$_4$/LTB$_5$	chemotaxis	+++/±
		neutrophil activation	+++/±
	PGE$_2$/PGE$_3$[2]	edemogenic	++/++
		nociception	++/?
		reduce TNFα, IL-1β;	++/?
	PGI$_2$/PGI$_3$	vasodilatation	+++/+++
		platelet aggregation	++/++
	TXA$_2$/TXA$_3$	vasoconstriction	+++/±
		platelet aggregation	+++/±
		increase TNFα, IL-lβ;	+/?

+++ = Very strong; ++ = strong; + = moderate; ± = weak or absent.
[1]Relative potency of homologous omega–6 and omega–3 eicosanoids.
[2]Little PGE$_3$ appears to be formed by cells in the presence of either endogenous or exogenous EPA.

EPA (C20:5omega–3) is the 20 carbon omega–3 homologue of AA and competes with AA for enzymatically mediated release from cell membranes and for metabolism by COX and terminal synthases. AA and EPA are also competitive substrates for 5-LO and the downstream enzymes that produce the 5-hydroxy fatty acids and leukotrienes, which are mediators of inflammation and allergy. In the presence of abundant dietary omega–3 fatty acids (especially omega–3 HUFA) and omega–6 PUFA, both omega–3 and omega–6 products of COX and 5-LO (collectively known as eicosanoids) will be formed. DHA (C22:6omega–3) is an omega–3 HUFA found with EPA in fish and fish oils. DHA can be converted to EPA and can also compete with AA.

The relative activities of omega–3 and omega–6 eicosanoids are important in determining the stability of homeostatic balance in response to physiological stressors, including inflammation. The relative potency of important activities of homologous omega–3 and omega–6 eicosanoids is summarized in table 1.

Since omega–3 eicosanoids are generally less pro-inflammatory or less prothrombotic than their omega–6 counterparts, it is to be expected that a diet hyperabundant in omega–6 PUFA and poor in omega–3 PUFA will favor a predilection for inflammatory diseases and adverse cardiovascular outcomes. While strong evidence exists for the latter, the evidence for the former is less abundant and less direct. However, the evidence that does exist generally supports this proposition. For example, in the Seattle Women's Health Study, the relative risk for seropositive rheumatoid arthritis in subjects consuming more than two fish meals per week was less than half that of subjects consuming less than one fish meal per week [7]. Also, Greenland Eskimo populations consuming their aboriginal diet have been shown to have a low frequency of inflammatory diseases, including rheumatoid arthritis [8]. They have also been observed to possess unusually high frequencies of the HLA alleles DRB1 0401, which is a risk factor for rheumatoid arthritis in other populations [9]. Although founder effects may exert the dominant influence, this association provides a basis for speculation about a possible interaction between an inflammation prone genotype and an environment where the diet, by virtue of abundance of omega–3 fats, has a propensity to reduce the intensity of inflammatory responses. According to this hypothesis, genotypes that strengthen specific immune responses to potential microbial pathogens may be especially advantageous within a setting where such responses are blunted by dietary dominance of omega–3 fats. By contrast, within the context of a pro-inflammatory omega–6 dominant diet, these same genetic factors may imbue an important predisposition to the emergence of the unwanted inflammation that characterized inflammatory diseases.

Effects of Dietary Omega–3 Fats on Inflammatory Cytokine Synthesis

Molvig reported stable interindividual differences in production of IL-1β and TNFα by monocytes from healthy subjects [10]. This observation suggested a genetically determined regulation of the rate of synthesis of these cytokines, which became apparent with the demonstration of a single base polymorphism in the TNFα promoter region which was a determinant of the extent of transcriptional activation of the TNFα gene [11, 12].

A number of studies have shown that dietary fortification with long chain omega–3 fats reduces the synthesis of IL-1β and TNFα by peripheral blood mononuclear cells (PBMC) in vitro [13–20]. However, some studies have failed to show these effects, which is not surprising given the variation between individuals in cytokine production [21–23]. However, recent investigations have shown that a polymorphism in the TNFβ (lymphotoxin) gene also is associated with different rates of PBMC TNFα synthesis and importantly, is associated with the response to dietary fish oil of TNFα synthesis [24]. These latter studies provide a basis for reconciling the positive and negative findings of earlier reports. Importantly, these genetic studies highlight the potential diversity in response to dietary change within genetically heterogeneous populations.

The observed effects of dietary omega–3 PUFA on IL-1β and TNFα synthesis are important because of the central role these cytokines play in orchestrating inflammatory responses. Their effects include upregulation of expression of proteolytic enzymes that degrade structural proteins in ways that can lead to tissue failure at sites of inflammation [5]. The importance of IL-1β and TNFα in mediating inflammatory diseases is underlined by the efficacy of biological agents designed to inhibit their effects in the treatment of chronic inflammatory diseases, such as rheumatoid arthritis [25–27]. Considering the extra-ordinary expense of these agents (typically in the order of USD 20,000 per patient per year), it is remarkable that no coordinated attempt has been made to combine inexpensive dietary omega–3 enrichment that has been shown to inhibit IL-1 and TNFα synthesis, with TNFα and IL-1β blockade. These differences in usage reflect the respective influences of resource intensive drug company marketing of proprietary agents on the one hand, and the relative ignorance and neglect by medical practitioners of rational nutritional approaches on the other.

Differences between Dietary Omega–3 Fats and NSAIDs

There are a number of important differences between dietary omega–3 supplements and NSAIDs that are important for implementation in the clinic. These differences are detailed in table 2.

Advantages of and Technique for Taking Bottled Fish Oil

A barrier to the implementation of fish oil treatment for inflammatory diseases has been the high cost and inconvenience of taking fish oil capsules in sufficient dosage to achieve an anti-inflammatory effect. For example, 10 capsules of standard fish oil capsules, containing 18% EPA and 12% DHA are required to achieve an intake of 3 g omega–3 LC PUFA daily. Fish oil concentrates (e.g. 30% EPA, 25% DHA) allow dose volumes to be reduced but at the expense of substantially increased cost. Bottled fish oil on juice in volumes of 10–20 ml can be ingested easily in a single swallow. A method for taking bottled fish oil juice that avoids the taste of fish at the time of ingestion and subsequent 'repeating' of the fish taste is shown in table 3.

Changes in Diet as a Complement to Omega–3 PUFA Ingestion
Choosing visible fats that are rich in monounsaturates with omega–3 α-linolenic acid (ALA, C18:3omega–3) (flaxseed oil, canola) or without ALA

Table 2. Differences between dietary omega–3 fats and NSAIDs relevant to clinical implementation

	Fish oil	NSAIDs
Time from introduction of therapy to symptomatic response	2–4 months depending on dose	<1 h
Toxicities	safe in doses up to 4 g daily (status of higher doses not known)	upper-GI events (bleeding, perforation) increased vascular risk (with rofecoxib)
Intolerance	taste, repeating	dyspepsia
Collateral health benefits	cardiovascular protective effect protection against ventricular arrythmias reduce atheroma formation in experimental models improve blood pressure control reduce renal toxicity of cyclosporin therapy improved outcomes in other inflammatory conditions (Crohn's disease, IgA nephropathy)	cardiovascular protective effect of low dose aspirin through unique irreversible inhibition of platelet COX-1

(olive oil) can enhance the tissue levels of omega–3 LC PUFA. The emphasis on monounsaturates allows avoidance of products based on omega–6 PUFA (sunflower, safflower, corn oils). The reduction of competitor omega–6 PUFA can enhance the conversion of ALA to EPA in vivo and can increase the uptake by tissues of dietary omega–3 LC PUFA [28–30] (fig. 3). Substitution of dietary omega–6 polyunsaturates for monounsaturates is a simple exercise for most people.

Rheumatoid Arthritis

Established rheumatoid arthritis (RA) presents an easily recognized and defined presentation that favors capture of relatively homogeneous groups of patients for clinical studies. Furthermore the pain and swelling of rheumatoid inflammation provide aspects of the condition that can be modified in the relatively short-term by anti-inflammatory agents. For these reasons, RA has

Table 3. Method for taking bottled fish oil that avoids direct and repeating taste

- Pour ~50 ml juice into a small to medium glass.
- Pour ~30 ml of juice into a smaller glass (e.g. a 'shot' or sherry glass). Layer the desired dose of fish oil onto the surface – do not stir. Pour with dominant hand.
- Using the dominant hand, bring the smaller glass containing the juice and oil into the mouth and swallow as a single gulp avoiding contact between the contents and the lips (where the oil can be tasted).
- Immediately follow with juice from the other glass. Hold this glass in the non dominant hand and sip slowly through the lips (to elute and mask the taste of any oil that may have reached the lips).
- The choice of juice is not critical – orange, tomato, vegetable and apple juices are acceptable. Cordial and any other strongly flavored drink can also be used. Avoid carbonated beverages, which by virtue of their gaseous content cause burping and 'repeating' of the fish taste.
- Take the dose immediately before undertaking oral hygiene and retiring to bed. Lie on the left side for at least 15 min to favor distribution of the oil to the passage from the stomach into the small intestine [54].
- Bottled fish body oils are preferable to cod liver oil since the latter can deliver undesirable amounts of vitamin A at anti-inflammatory doses.
- Bottled fish oil should be kept refrigerated after opening.

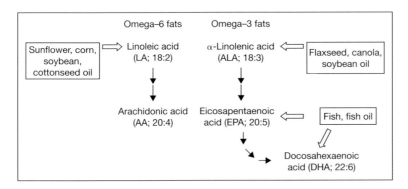

Fig. 3. Metabolism of 18-carbon fatty acids to longer chain fatty acids.

been used extensively to test various treatment regimens, including fish oil. To date there have been at least thirteen randomized controlled trials of fish oil in late rheumatoid arthritis (summarized in table 4). All have shown symptomatic benefit, with almost all studies showing reduced pain and morning stiffness. Typically, the improvement is seen after a delay of two to four months.

Table 4. Summary of salient findings from studies of fish oil in rheumatoid arthritis

Study	Number of subjects for analysis	Treatment periods weeks	Medication	Omega–3 fat supplement g/day	Outcome measures which improved significantly in the fish oil group
Kremer et al. [55]	38	12	continued	1.8 g EPA 1.2 g DHA	number of tender joints, duration of morning stiffness
Kremer et al. [56]	33	14	continued	2.7 g EPA 1.8 g DHA	ARA class, physician's global assessment, no. of tender joints, number of swollen joints, time to fatigue
Cleland et al. [57]	46	12	continued	3.2 g EPA 2.0 g DHA	number of tender joints, grip strength
Kremer et al. [20]	49	24	continued (change was a withdrawal criterion)	low dose: 1.7 g EPA, 1.2 g DHA or high dose: 3.5 g EPA, 2.4 g DHA	number of swollen joints, number of tender joints, grip strength, physician's global assessment, duration of morning stiffness (high dose only)
Tulleken et al. [58]	27	12	continued	2.0 g EPA 1.3 g DHA	number of swollen joints, joint pain index
van der Tempel et al. [59]	14	12	continued	2.0 g EPA 1.3 g DHA	number of swollen joints, duration of morning stiffness
Skoldstam et al. [60]	43	24	continued SAARD free to change NSAID	1.8 g EPA 1.2 g DHA	physician global assessment, no. and severity of tender joints (Ritchie Index), decreased NSAID use.
Kjeldsen-Kragh et al. [61]	67	16	continued SAARD. NSAID continued in group A and stopped at 10 weeks in group B	3.8 g EPA 2.0 g DHA	number and severity of tender joints (Ritchie Index), duration of morning stiffness

Table 4 (continued)

Study	Number of subjects for analysis	Treatment periods weeks	Medication	Omega–3 fat supplement g/day	Outcome measures which improved significantly in the fish oil group
Nielsen et al. [62]	51	12	continued (change was a withdrawal criterion)	2.0 g EPA 1.2 g DHA	duration of morning stiffness, no of tender joints, C-reactive protein levels
Lau et al. [63]	64 at entry[1]	52	none on SAARD; change in NSAIDs was the end-point	1.7 g EPA, 1.1 g DHA	reduced NSAID use
Geusens et al. [64]	60	52	varied as required during study	low dose: 0.86 g EPA, 0.18 g DHA or high dose: 1.7 g EPA, 0.36 g DHA	physician pain assessment, patient global assessment, and decreased NSAID and/or SAARD use (high dose only)
Kremer et al. [65]	49	26 or 30	continued SAARD and NSAID, but NSAID was stopped at 18 or 22 weeks	4.6 g EPA, 2.5 g DHA[2]	number of tender joints, duration of morning stiffness, physician pain assessment, physician and patient global assessment (all at 18 or 22 weeks)
Volker et al. [66]	26	15	continued (change was a withdrawal criterion); linoleic acid intake was <10 g/day	1.3 g EPA, 1.0 g DHA[2]	within group: swollen joint count, morning stiffness, pain score, physician and patient global assessment, HAQ; between groups: morning stiffness, HAQ

EPA = Eicosapentaenoic acid; DHA = docosahexaenoic acid; NSAID = non-steroidal anti-inflammatory drug; SAARD = slow-acting anti-rheumatic drug.

[1]Variable; numbers had dropped at each 3-monthly assessment over a 15-month period.

[2]Based on 65-kg subjects.

In a study in which two doses of fish oil and a vegetable oil were compared, the time to improvement with fish oil was less with the higher fish oil dose [20]. The ultimate symptomatic effect of the lower dose was similar to that of the higher dose. These data suggest that a higher load dose followed by a lower maintenance dose could be the most efficient approach to fish oil treatment in RA, although further studies are needed to address this issue more fully.

Important unanswered questions include the possible long-term beneficial effects of dietary omega–3 fats on outcomes in RA. One possible but unproven benefit is reduced joint damage since dietary supplementation with fish oils has been shown to reduce synthesis of IL-1β and TNFα, which up regulate release of the proteolytic enzymes that mediate tissue damage in RA [31]. A further potential benefit is reduced risk for cardiovascular events for which subjects with RA are especially prone [32, 33] and for which dietary omega–3 fats have been observed to be protective [34]. Another important unaddressed issue is the place of dietary omega–3 enrichment in general and fish oil supplements in particular with multiple drug regimens now used for treatment of recent onset RA [35]. This latter issue is especially important as early diagnosis and treatment and use of combinations of long-acting anti-rheumatic drugs have been shown to provide substantially improved responses to treatment. In studies of fish oil in RA, genotyping could prove important, since genetic factors may been associated with levels of production of TNFα in vitro and response to dietary fish oil supplements [24]. As discussed above, dietary omega–3 PUFA may have a preventive effect against RA [7] but more direct evidence is needed.

Osteoarthritis

A potential for benefit of dietary fish oil in osteoarthritis has been suggested by studies showing an inhibitory effect of omega–3 HUFA on release by IL-1β treated cartilage explants of catabolic enzymes that mediate cartilage damage [36]. Surprisingly no clinical trials into the effects of fish oil in osteoarthritis have been reported. By extrapolation from studies of fish oil in RA, symptomatic benefit, if present, could be delayed several months from the onset of treatment.

Gout

In the early 18th and early 19th Centuries, the use of cod liver oil in the treatment of gout was reported [37]. The beneficial effects described are consistent with the subsequently determined anti-inflammatory effects of omega–3 HUFA found in fish oils. No studies of fish oil in gout appear to have been undertaken in the modern era. Possible benefits include reduced tendency to acute attacks, which could be especially useful in the troublesome phase of aggravation of attacks that occurs during the induction phase of long-term hypouricemic therapy. This problem is thought to relate to mobilization of existent urate deposits, which as a result of partial dissolution may become especially prone to release into joints, where their irritant properties cause the attacks of inflammation that characterize acute gout.

Seronegative Spondyloarthritis

There is a paucity of data regarding the possible benefits of fish oils in seronegative spondyloarthritis. The important pathological distinction between these arthropathies and RA is their propensity for entheseal involvement in spondyloarthritis (an enthesis is the site of insertion of a ligament or tendon into bone). However, apart from this peculiarity, the inflammation of spondylo-arthritis resembles that of RA, both in terms of participant cells and mediators and general response to anti-inflammatory agents. A further basis for optimism regarding the possible benefit of fish oil in spondyloarthritis is the reported benefit seen with fish oil in inflammatory conditions with which they are asso-ciated, such as psoriasis [38], Crohn's disease [39] and IgA nephropathy [40].

Omega–3 PUFA – Drug Interactions

There are a number of ways in which dietary fish oil supplements may interact favorably with anti-inflammatory drugs. Fish oil supplements have been shown to reduce NSAID requirements in RA [32]. Since NSAIDs have not been shown to improve long-term outcomes in any form of arthritis, their displacement by a nutritional factor that has collateral cardiovascular health benefits and no evident toxicities should be an advantage.

While omega–6 eicosanoids are generally regarded as pro-inflammatory, it has become apparent that anti-inflammatory omega–6 and omega–3 eicosanoids can be produced also and that their production may be increased in the resolu-tion phase of inflammation and may be assisted by aspirin [41, 42]. While aspirin inhibits prostaglandin production via both COX-1 and COX-2, the acetylation by aspirin of the ser-516 residue in the active site of COX-2 results in formation of 15R-hydroxy eicosatetraenoic acid (15R-HETE) from AA [43]. 15R-HETE is a substrate for 5-lipoxygenase formation of the trihydroxy epi-lipoxins, 15-epi-LXA$_4$ and 15-epi-LXB$_4$, which have anti-inflammatory properties [44]. In addition, EPA and DHA are converted by a similar route first involving aspirin-treated COX-2 followed by leukocyte 5-lipoxygenase activity to produce tri-hydroxy eicosapentaenoic acids (HEPEs) and tri-hydroxy DHA derivatives all of which are anti-inflammatory in the murine air pouch model [41, 42]. Thus, careful lipid analyses are revealing cooperativity between aspirin and fatty acids to form a hitherto unrecognized group of anti-inflammatory compounds.

While highly selective COX-2 inhibitors relieve the signs and symptoms of inflammation, they may increase risk for serious adverse cardiovascular events by disturbing balance between the homeostatic action of TXA_2 and PGI_2 in the vascular space since they inhibit COX-2-derived PGI_2 synthesis selectively without influencing COX-1-derived platelet TXA_2 production [45]. This effect is likely to be ameliorated by the inhibitory effect of EPA on TXA_2 synthesis. The overall cardioprotective effects of omega–3 LC PUFA are also likely to run counter to the potentially increased risk accompanying the homocyteinemia that has been associated with methotrexate and sulphasalazine, especially when, as is commonly the case, they are give in combination [46]. This effect on blood homocysteine levels is likely to be associated with the interference of these drugs with metabolism of folate [47, 48], which has an important influence on homocysteine metabolism [49]. Homocysteinemia is a risk factor for vascular disease to which rheumatoid subjects are especially prone [33], possibly through its capacity to cause endothelial cell activation, a process that has been shown to be increased by omega–6 linoleic acid and to be inhibited by omega–3 PUFA [50].

Glucocorticoid therapy can also increase risk for cardiovascular events [51] against which omega–3 PUFA may likewise provide protection. Glucocorticoid therapy can also cause osteoporosis [51]. Dietary omega–3 PUFA supplements have been shown to increase bone density [52]. The effect of fish oil supplements on glucocorticoid-induced osteoporosis has not been reported. Fish oil supplements have been shown to ameliorate the nephrotoxicity and hypertension that occurs commonly with cyclosporin A therapy [53].

Finally, since fish oil supplements have been shown to reduce IL-1β and TNFα synthesis, it would be rational to evaluate their use in combination with the highly expensive biological agents that have been designed to block the action of these cytokines.

Conclusion

In conclusion, individuals can make food choices that determine a broad range of reciprocally related omega–6 and omega–3 HUFA in their tissues. While choices are conditioned by cultural factors, in developed countries where omega–6 dominance of PUFA in the diet is most prevalent, relatively simple food choices can be made to reduce omega–6 PUFA and to replace them with monounsaturates and omega–3 PUFA which are not precursors of pro-inflammatory eicosanoids. The greater efficiency of ingestion of EPA and DHA for increasing tissue omega–3 HUFA levels, makes fish and fish oils especially useful in reducing production of omega–6 derived inflammatory eicosanoids. Omega–3 dietary enrichment may potentially reduce risk for development of certain types of arthritis, as well as helping to provide relief from arthritis when it occurs. Additionally, dietary omega–3 fats may have collateral benefits in rheumatoid arthritis by reducing the disease-associated increased cardiovascular risk. While EPA + DHA intakes of 3 g daily may be needed for anti-inflammatory effects, substantially lower doses will provide cardiovascular protection.

References

1   Lands WEM, Libelt B, Morris A, et al: Maintenance of lower proportions of (n-6) eicosanoid precursors in phospholipids of human plasma in response to added dietary (n-3) fatty acids. Biochim Biophys Acta 1992;1180:147–162.
2   James MJ, Cleland LG, Rofe AM, Leslie AL: Intraarticular pressure and the relationship between synovial perfusion and metabolic demand. J Rheumatol 1990;17:521–527.
3   Moncada S, Ferreira SH, Vane JR: Inhibition of prostaglandin biosynthesis as the mechanism of analgesia of aspirin-like drugs in the dog knee joint. Eur J Pharmacol 1975;31:250–260.
4   Caughey GE, Pouliot M, Cleland LG, James MJ: Regulation of tumor necrosis factor alpha and interleukin-1 beta synthesis by thromboxane A_2 in non-adherent human monocytes. J Immunol 1997;158:351–358.
5   Westacott CI, Sharif M: Cytokines in osteoarthritis: mediators or markers of joint destruction? Semin Arthritis Rheum 1996;25:254–272.
6   Penglis PS, Cleland LG, Demasi M, Caughey GE, James MJ: Differential regulation of prostaglandin E_2 and thromboxane A_2 production in human monocytes: Implications for the use of cyclooxygenase inhibitors. J Immunol 2000;165:1605–1611.
7   Shapiro JA, Koepsell TD, Voigt LF, Dugowson CE, Kestin M, Nelson JL: Diet and rheumatoid arthritis in women: A possible protective effect of fish consumption. Epidemiology 1996;7:256–263.
8   Harvald B: Genetic epidemiology of Greenland. Clin Genet 1989;36:364–367.
9   Welinder L, Graugaard B, Madsen M: HLA antigen and gene frequencies in Eskimos of East Greenland. Eur J Immunogenet 2000;27:93–97.
10 Molvig J, Baek L, Christensen P, et al: Endotoxin-stimulated human monocyte secretion of interleukin 1, tumour necrosis factor alpha, and prostaglandin E2 shows stable interindividual differences. Scand J Immunol 1988;27:705–716.
11 Wilson AG, di Giovine FS, Blakemore AI, Duff GW: Single base polymorphism in the human tumour necrosis factor alpha (TNF alpha) gene detectable by NcoI restriction of PCR product. Hum Mol Genet 1992;1:353.
12 Wilson AG, Symons JA, McDowell TL, McDevitt HO, Duff GW: Effects of a polymorphism in the human tumor necrosis factor alpha promoter on transcriptional activation. Proc Natl Acad Sci USA 1997;94:3195–3199.
13 Endres S, Ghorbani R, Kelley VE, et al: The effect of dietary supplementation with n-3 polyunsaturated fatty acids on the synthesis of interleukin-1 and tumor necrosis factor by mononuclear cells. N Engl J Med 1989;320:265–271.

14   Meydani S, Endres S, Woods MM, et al: Oral (n-3) fatty acid supplementation suppresses cytokine production and lymphocyte proliferation: comparison between younger and older women. J Nutr 1991;121:547–555.

15   Caughey GE, Mantzioris E, Gibson RA, Cleland LG, James MJ: The effect on human tumor necrosis factor-a and interleukin-1b production of diets enriched in n-3 fatty acids from vegetable oil or fish oil. Am J Clin Nutr 1996;63:116–122.

16   Gallai V, Sarchielli P, Trequattrini A, et al: Cytokine secretion and eicosanoid production in the peripheral blood mononuclear cells of MS patients undergoing dietary supplementation with n-3 polyunsaturated fatty acids. J Neuroimmunol 1995;56:143–153.

17   Cooper AL, Gibbons L, Horan MA, Little RA, Rothwell NJ: Effect of dietary fish oil supplementation on fever and cytokine production in human volunteers. Clin Nutr 1993;12:321–328.

18   Kelley DS, Taylor PC, Nelson GJ, et al: Docosahexaenoic acid ingestion inhibits natural killer cell activity and production of inflammatory mediators in young healthy men. Lipids 1999;34:317–324.

19   Meydani SN, Lichtenstein AH, Cornwall S, et al: Immunologic effects of National Cholesterol Education Panel Step-2 diets with and without fish-derived n-3 fatty acid enrichment. J Clin Invest 1993;92:105–113.

20   Kremer JM, Lawrence DA, Jubiz W, et al: Dietary fish oil and olive oil supplementation in patients with rheumatoid arthritis. Arthritis Rheum 1990;33:810–820.

21   Schmidt EB, Varming K, Moller JM, Pedersen BI, Madsen P, Dyerberg J: No effect of a very low dose of n-3 fatty acids on monocyte function in healthy humans. Scand J Clin Lab Invest 1996; 56:87–92.

22   Blok WL, Deslypere JP, Demacker PN, et al: Pro- and anti-inflammatory cytokines in healthy volunteers fed various doses of fish oil for 1 year. Eur J Clin Invest 1997;27:1003–1008.

23   Molvig J, Pociot F, Worsaae H, et al: Dietary supplementation with omega–3-polyunsaturated fatty acids decreases mononuclear cell proliferation and interleukin-1 beta content but not monokine secretion in healthy and insulin-dependent diabetic individuals. Scand J Immunol 1991;34: 399–410.

24   Grimble RF, Howell WM, O'Reilly G, et al: The ability of fish oil to suppress tumor necrosis factor alpha production by peripheral blood mononuclear cells in healthy men is associated with polymorphisms in genes that influence tumor necrosis factor alpha production. Am J Clin Nutr 2002;76:454–459.

25   Arend WP: The mode of action of cytokine inhibitors. J Rheumatol 2002;29:16–21.

26   Bresnihan B: Preventing joint damage as the best measure of biologic drug therapy. J Rheumatol Suppl 2002;65:39–43.

27   Cohen SB, Woolley JM, Chan W: Interleukin 1 receptor antagonist anakinra improves functional status in patients with rheumatoid arthritis. J Rheumatol 2003;30:225–231.

28   Emken EA, Adlof RO, Gulley RM: Dietary linoleic acid influences desaturation and acylation of deuterium-labeled linoleic and linolenic acids in young adult males. Biochim Biophys Acta 1994; 1213:277–288.

29   Cleland LG, James MJ, Neumann MA, D'Angelo M, Gibson RA: Linoleate inhibits EPA incorporation from dietary fish oil supplements in human subjects. Am J Clin Nutr 1992;55:395–399.

30   Mantzioris E, James MJ, Gibson RA, Cleland LG: Dietary substitution with an a-linolenic acid-rich vegetable oil increases eicosapentaenoic acid concentrations in tissues. Am J Clin Nutr 1994;59:1304–1309.

31   James MJ, Cleland LG: Dietary n-3 fatty acids and therapy for rheumatoid arthritis. Semin Arthritis Rheum 1997;27:85–97.

32   Cleland LG, James MJ: Fish oil and rheumatoid arthritis: Anti-inflammatory and collateral health benefits. J Rheumatol 2000;27:2305–2307.

33   Bacon PA, Townend JN: Nail in the coffin: Increasing evidence for the role of rheumatic disease in the cardiovascular mortality of rheumatoid arthritis. Arthritis Rheum 2001;44:2707–2710.

34   O'Keefe JH Jr, Harris WS: From Inuit to implementation: omega–3 fatty acids come of age. Mayo Clin Proc 2000;75:607–614.

35   Emery P, Breedveld FC, Dougados M, Kalden JR, Schiff MH, Smolen JS: Early referral recommendation for newly diagnosed rheumatoid arthritis: Evidence based development of a clinical guide. Ann Rheum Dis 2002;61:290–297.

36 Curtis CL, Rees SG, Little CB, et al: Pathologic indicators of degradation and inflammation in human osteoarthritic cartilage are abrogated by exposure to n-3 fatty acids. Arthritis Rheum 2002; 46:1544–1553.

37 de Jongh LJ: Cod Liver Oil: Chemical and Therapeutic Properties (translated by Taylor CE). London, Walton, Maberly, 1849.

38 Mayser P, Mrowietz U, Arenberger P, et al: Omega–3 fatty acid-based lipid infusion in patients with chronic plaque psoriasis: Results of a double-blind, randomized, placebo-controlled, multi-center trial. J Am Acad Dermatol 1998;38:539–547.

39 Belluzzi A, Brignola C, Campieri M, Pera A, Boschi S, Miglioli M: Effect of an enteric-coated fish-oil preparation on relapses in Crohn's disease. N Engl J Med 1996;334:1557–1560.

40 Donadio JV: The emerging role of omega–3 polyunsaturated fatty acids in the management of patients with IgA nephropathy. J Ren Nutr 2001;11:122–128.

41 Serhan CN, Clish CB, Brannon J, Colgan SP, Chiang N, Gronert K: Novel functional sets of lipid-derived mediators with antiinflammatory actions generated from omega–3 fatty acids via cyclooxygenase-2 nonsteroidal antiinflammatory drugs and transcellular processing. J Exp Med 2000;192:1197–1204.

42 Serhan CN, Hong S, Gronert K, et al: Resolvins: A family of bioactive products of omega–3 fatty acid transformation circuits initiated by aspirin treatment that counter proinflammation signals. J Exp Med 2002;196:1025–1037.

43 Lecomte M, Laneuville O, Ji C, DeWitt DL, Smith WL: Acetylation of human prostaglandin endoperoxide synthase-2 (cyclooxygenase-2) by aspirin. J Biol Chem 1994;269:13207–13215.

44 Serhan CN, Oliw E: Unorthodox routes to prostanoid formation: New twists in cyclooxygenase-initiated pathways. J Clin Invest 2001;107:1481–1489.

45 Cleland LG, James MJ, Stamp LK, Penglis PS: COX-2 inhibition and thrombotic tendency: a need for surveillance. Med J Aust 2001;175:214–217.

46 Haagsma CJ, Blom HJ, van Riel PL, et al: Influence of sulphasalazine, methotrexate, and the combination of both on plasma homocysteine concentrations in patients with rheumatoid arthritis. Ann Rheum Dis 1999;58:79–84.

47 Kumagai K, Hiyama K, Oyama T, Maeda H, Kohno N: Polymorphisms in the thymidylate syn-thase and methylenetetrahydrofolate reductase genes and sensitivity to the low-dose methotrexate therapy in patients with rheumatoid arthritis. Int J Mol Med 2003;11:593–600.

48 Baggott JE, Morgan SL, Ha T, Vaughn WH, Hine RJ: Inhibition of folate-dependent enzymes by non-steroidal anti-inflammatory drugs. Biochem J 1992;282:197–202.

49 Selhub J, Jacques PF, Wilson PW, Rush D, Rosenberg IH: Vitamin status and intake as primary determinants of homocysteinemia in an elderly population. JAMA 1993;270:2693–2698.

50 Dichtl W, Ares MP, Jonson AN, et al: Linoleic acid-stimulated vascular adhesion molecule-1 expression in endothelial cells depends on nuclear factor-kappaB activation. Metabolism 2002;51: 327–333.

51 Frauman AG: An overview of the adverse reactions to adrenal corticosteroids. Adverse Drug React Toxicol Rev 1996;15:203–206.

52 Kruger MC, Coetzer H, de Winter R, Gericke G, van Papendorp DH: Calcium, gamma-linolenic acid and eicosapentaenoic acid supplementation in senile osteoporosis. Aging (Milano) 1998;10:385–394.

53 Darlametsos IE, Varonos DD: Role of prostanoids and endothelins in the prevention of cyclosporine-induced nephrotoxicity. Prostagl Leukotr Essential Fatty Acids 2001;64:231–239.

54 Horowitz M, Jones K, Edelbroek MA, Smout AJ, Read NW: The effect of posture on gastric empty-ing and intragastric distribution of oil and aqueous meal components and appetite. Gastroenterology 1993;105:382–390.

55 Kremer JM, Bigauoette J, Michalek AV, et al: Effects of manipulation of dietary fatty acids on clinical manifestations of rheumatoid arthritis. Lancet 1985;i:184–187.

56 Kremer JM, Jubiz W, Michalek A, et al: Fish-oil fatty acid supplementation in active rheumatoid arthritis. Ann Intern Med 1987;106:497–503.

57 Cleland LG, French JK, Betts WH, Murphy GA, Elliott M: Clinical and biochemical effects of dietary fish oil supplements in rheumatoid arthritis. J Rheumatol 1988;15:1471–1475.

58 Tulleken JE, Limburg PC, Muskiet FAJ, van Rijswijk MH: Vitamin E status during dietary fish oil supplementation in rheumatoid arthritis. Arthritis Rheum 1990;33:1416–1419.

59   van der Tempel H, Tulleken JE, Limburg PC, Muskiet FAJ, van Rijswijk MH: Effects of fish oil supplementation in rheumatoid arthritis. Ann Rheum Dis 1990;49:76–80.

60   Skoldstam L, Borjesson O, Kjallman A, Seiving B, Akesson B: Effect of six months of fish oil supplementation in stable rheumatoid arthritis: A double blind, controlled study. Scand J Rheumatol 1992;21:178–185.

61   Kjeldsen-Kragh J, Lund JA, Riise T, et al: Dietary omega–3 fatty acid supplementation and naproxen treatment in patients with rheumatoid arthritis. J Rheumatol 1992;19:1531–1536.

62   Nielsen GL, Faarvang KL, Thomsen BS, et al: The effects of dietary supplementation with n-3 polyunsaturated fatty acids in patients with rheumatoid arthritis: a randomized double blind trial. Eur J Clin Invest 1992;22:687–691.

63   Lau CS, Morley KD, Belch JJF: Effects of fish oil supplementation on non-steroidal anti-inflammatory drug requirement in patients with mild rheumatoid arthritis – a double blind placebo controlled study. Br J Rheumatol 1993;32:982–989.

64   Geusens P, Wouters C, Nijs J, Jiang Y, Dequeker J: Long-term effect of omega–3 fatty acid supplementation in active rheumatoid arthritis. Arthritis Rheum 1994;37:824–829.

65   Kremer JM, Lawrence DA, Petrillo GF, et al: Effects of high-dose fish oil on rheumatoid arthritis after stopping nonsteroidal antiinflammatory drugs. Arthritis Rheum 1995;38:1107–1114.

66   Volker D, Fitzgerald P, Major G, Garg M: Efficacy of fish oil concentrate in the treatment of rheumatoid arthritis. J Rheumatol 2000;27:2343–2346.

Prof. Leslie G. Cleland
Rheumatology Unit, Royal Adelaide Hospital
North Terrace, 5000 Adelaide, S.A. (Australia)
Tel. +1 8 8222 5190, Fax +1 8 8222 5895, E-Mail lcleland@mail.rah.sa.gov.au

Author Index

Subject Index